Doctor Solomon's
Proven Master Plan For Total Body Fitness And Maintenance

Also by Dr. Solomon:

DR. SOLOMON'S
EASY NO-RISK DIET

Doctor Solomon's
Proven Master Plan For Total Body Fitness And Maintenance

by
Dr. Neil Solomon
and
Evalee Harrison

G. P. PUTNAM'S SONS,
NEW YORK

Copyright © 1976 by Dr. Neil Solomon and Evalee Harrison

All rights reserved. This book, or parts thereof, must not be reproduced in any form without permission. Published on the same day in Canada by Longman Canada Limited, Toronto.

SBN: 399-11591-9

Library of Congress Cataloging in Publication Data
Solomon, Neil, 1932-
   Doctor Solomon's personalized, common sense exercise plan for total body therapy.

   Bibliography: p.
   1. Exercise. I. Title. [DNLM: 1. Physical fitness. 2. Gymnastics. QT255 S689d]
RA781.S623 1976   613.7'1   75-43745

Photos © by William Douglas Ganslen, San Francisco
PRINTED IN THE UNITED STATES OF AMERICA

Dedication

Neil Solomon: I dedicate this book to my loving, talented, and patient wife, Frema, who is my first choice as wife, mistress, and mother of my children.

Without her, I could not have been blessed with my three wonderful sons, Ted, Scott, and Cliff, who along with Frema make me very, very happy.

Evalee Harrison: I dedicate this book to Dr. Sheldon Margen, whose creativity, understanding, and thoughtfulness have helped me through many troubled times; he has been a continuing inspiration to me.

Neil Solomon and Evalee Harrison: We dedicate this book to our mother, Clara, and our father, Max, who gave us the love and understanding to help others.

Contents

Preface	9
Foreword	11

PART I

1	The Why and the How and the Promise	17
2	Alternative Programs: The Perils of Fad Exercise	24
3	All About You: Defining Your Own Needs	36

PART II

4	Priming for Exercise	49
5	The Master Plan	55

PART III

6	Area of Concentration: The Abdomen	75
7	Area of Concentration: The Arms and Chest	83
8	Area of Concentration: The Back	90
9	Area of Concentration: The Buttocks	99

	10 Area of Concentration: The Feet and Ankles	106
	11 Area of Concentration: The Hips	112
	12 Area of Concentration: The Legs, Knees, and Thighs	122
	13 Area of Concentration: The Waistline and Midriff	131

PART IV

	14 Coping with Fatigue	141
	15 Back Pain: Helpful Exercises	145
	16 On the Road	152
	17 Family Fitness	157
	18 Sexual Fitness for Men and Women	165
	19 Exercising Eating Awareness	176
	20 Movement Therapy	181
	21 How to Relax	186

Afterword	190
Glossary	191

Preface

Will you give a little to get a lot? Are you willing to try a few new things? If your answer is yes, and you are willing to think about yourself a little differently and do a little more each day, then this book can maximize what you have going for you. It can lead you to a new awareness of your body and the way you move it that will make each day more pleasurable.

If you are in poor physical shape, this book will help you to attain a better level of physical fitness. If you are now in good physical condition, it will show you how to maintain this with a minimum of effort. If you feel old, it will help you to add new zest to your life with exercise. You will live longer and look younger. If you are young, the book will help you develop the sort of personal exercise program that will enable you to keep fit as long as you live.

The beauty of exercise is that there is no other aid to good health that is as inexpensive, as available to everyone, and as easy to do. We hope that in this book we can pique your interest and involve you in a new commitment to yourself and your future well-being.

Our program has been tested by more than 5,000 people, ranging in age from six to ninety-four years and drawn from a cross-cultural group of whites, blacks, Asians, and Hispanics. It has worked for them. It can work for you.

Foreword

In twelve years of private practice, after seeing and helping more than 5,000 obese patients, I can safely say that I have never treated exactly the same problem twice. Each patient has had to be handled as an individual—diagnosed and treated as such. Only one factor held true for just about all of those 5,000 individuals: they simply did not exercise enough. The problem was, and is, to get them moving.

Because I like to keep all of my own problems within the family, I consulted with my sister, Evalee Harrison, who is an expert in the field of body awareness and fitness. Evalee is currently a staff research associate in the Department of Nutritional Sciences at the University of California at Berkeley. She has worked with teenagers, women (both homemakers and those who worked outside the home), and men for more than fifteen years, evolving an exercise technique that is enjoyable and successful. Pooling our talents, we have designed an exercise plan which we have found to be beneficial to everyone who followed it, and, at the same time, easily adaptable to special and individual needs.

Did it make a difference to my patients? The results were renewed vigor and uplifted spirits. Almost all of them report that they are happier and healthier people today, and they definitely look better. The only thing that has changed in their lives—aside from their attitude—is *movement*. They do a lot more of it; and because they do, their attitudes toward exercise have done an about-face. Once I could not drive them to exercise; now they tell me they'll be exercising the rest of their lives.

If it works for 5,000, why not extend the benefits to as many more as possible? One group weight-control organization, the Diet Workshop, has incorporated elements of the plan into its new Body Design program, soon to be adapted by its exercise consultant for use in the workshop groups as an advanced exercise program.

The next logical step seemed to be this book, where we combined my research in endocrinology and metabolism and my experience with patients with Evalee's activities in physical fitness and client studies. We think we have evolved a fitness guide that is not only sound from each of our standpoints but also practical for the reader. We hope that you agree.

To all the physicians, physical therapists, and others in the exercising professions who have given their time to read and criticize our manuscript, a sincere thank you.

For his sincere interest and redoubtable suggestions, we thank Clyde C. Taylor, publisher of G. P. Putnam's Sons. His encouragement and confidence have been major assets. We appreciate also the excellent editorial assistance of Mildred Sindell and Paula Hummel. My warm gratitude to my wife, Frema, for her common sense and womanly touches. Thanks also to our two nurse sisters, Beverly Willner and Miriam Glazer, for their tips and moral support. My thanks also to Beatrice Wang, Rona Kogan, and Patricia Susan Hosey, who gave yeoman service and devotion in helping type this manuscript.

To all devotees of our systems—patients and clients alike—and the unknown but welcome readers of my diet books who prodded us along, thank you. Every one of you merits our friendly indebtedness. We are truly grateful.

Part I

1 The Why and the How and the Promise

What do people mean when they say they want to lose weight? On a conscious level, they mean just what they say. They want those pounds to disappear. I know because of the mail I received after my recent book, *Dr. Solomon's Easy No-Risk Diet,* written with medical writer Mary Knudson. By multiplying the number of letters and the weight losses reported, tons of fat have disappeared from the American scene.

This should mean that all of the writers were unqualifiedly happy. All had said they wanted to lose weight. Those who wrote, wrote to report success. Yet, in many of the letters the unspoken message behind "I want to lose weight" was finally brought out into the open. What people want to go along with weight loss is a better appearance.

"The pounds are gone, but I still don't like my silhouette."

"I'm thinner, not trimmer."

"Help! I'm still flabby!"

Dr. Jean Mayer, the noted nutritionist, was the first to call attention to the reassuring knowledge that sedentary people who increased their activity actually ate less and reduced even more easily. There is a double benefit to exercise, because it burns calories and at the same time decreases the number of calories consumed.

At this point, I stopped acting solo and brought in my sister as my consultant. Out of that consultation has come this book, because Evalee had already placed many of her California exercise clients on my diet program. They were happy and trimmer. I took her exercises and adapted them for my obesity patients, with dramatic and satisfying results.

Now this patient group is a broad spectrum. I have patients who are age six, and at the other end of the scale, I have a patient of ninety-four. The fat is distributed between males and females. Tailoring the exercises to specific needs, we watched the group carefully. In only a few months, caliper tests proved conclusively that there had been a loss of subcutaneous fat.

What especially pleased me was that those who had arrived on my doorstep as self-diagnosed "cellulite" problems were themselves pleased. Fat is fat, whether you translate it into French and call it "cellulite" or face the fact in English with a succinct three-letter word. French and fancy, or plain and English, there is no difference in the type of fat; it is that ugly stuff that accumulates under your skin and distributes itself across your body in unattractive patterns. The women, in particular, who complained to me about their "cellulite" happily discovered that moving around in a series of carefully designed exercises destroyed those bulges in the buttocks, the hips, and the thighs when they were also faithful to the diet. In fact, those who did not reduce discovered that their appearance improved anyway!

The Why and the How and the Promise

Why is exercise so important? And why are people so suddenly interested in it?

First of all, the evidence is building that exercise benefits everyone—from babies through the senior-citizen set. (The seniors who are exercising are certainly not going to become passive senior citizens!) While we have learned that exercise is for all ages, as a society we have cut ourselves off from moving around much physically after the age of twenty-five. As a consequence, flab develops, tension and muscle tone decrease to the point where atrophy or wasting results. Once muscle atrophy sets in, movements are restricted. When movements are restricted, more flab develops, the muscle tone decreases; and there you are, caught on a motionless merry-go-round from which you can't get off!

If we begin to decrease our exercise at age twenty-five, correspondingly we fail to decrease our caloric intake. On into middle age, we continue to eat like adolescents. We fast-food it for lunch, load up on drinks and desserts, and totally ignore the fact that after thirty we require about 1 percent fewer calories each year. We sit in our comfortable grooves, moving only the same small group of muscles through repetitive patterns of action, day after day and year after year, overlooking the fact that there are approximately 639 muscles in the body, not to mention 208 bones, and that all of them should be given the opportunity for a little fun and motion every twenty-four hours.

Put it all together, and you come up with one fact: *Overall exercise is necessary for each one of us.* We must compensate those muscles we neglect in our daily lives, we must firm up the muscles that have been neglected by disuse, we must burn up more calories to make up for our lowered calorie requirements, and we must keep moving just to maintain freedom of movement.

You might think that this would be reason enough for a great stir among the populace. But it isn't. For everyone who should exercise, there is a reason not to exercise. "I want exercises that are pleasant and easy to do," is the most common one. "I like to set my own pace," is another. "I'd kill myself if I did anything that strenuous or fatiguing," is a third. Finally, and with complete dismissal in the voice, there is the ultimate reason not to exercise: "The results aren't fast enough. There has to be an easier way." No wonder one out of three Americans is still considered out of condition or obese.

The fact is that exercise, of and by itself, can elevate the mood; it's a true upper! A good exercise program leaves the exerciser less tired, rather than fatigued, as the popular view would have it. And while you are making yourself feel emotionally and physically relaxed by exercising, you are achieving measurable and desirable side effects in the form of good health and physically fit bodies.

Let's talk about some of these side effects, a horrible term that sounds dangerous in most cases. However, the side effects of exercise remove dangers. The unique program of total body therapy you will find in this book provides you with an easy way to exercise. At the same time, as a side effect, it should help avoid premature aging and provide you with a general feeling of well-being.

Try it for fifteen minutes a day, at least three days a week, preferably four, but ideally every day. This program is enough for a more desirable level of health and fitness. It will also help with weight control, increase your energy output, improve your circulation, perhaps lower your cholesterol, put new zip into your sex life, and—if that doesn't motivate you enough—help prevent disease.

Are you suffering from maxi-proportion, mini-lethargy, body boredom? Now is the time to begin to fashion yourself into a new image with our exercises. We can add some enjoyment to your life—not with magic formulas, because an abracadabra won't work. The work belongs to you, but it is the kind of work that is fun while you are doing it and rewarding as it progresses. We'll route you through a choice of programs that other people have loved doing. None of the exercises are too time-consuming; they are varied, and far from monotonous. Results will come—and quickly enough to satisfy you physically and aesthetically.

You begin *not* on the exercise pad, but with some initial exploration of yourself so that you will understand and be able to plan intelligently how, why, and when you wish to exercise.

Perhaps you are already "into" some other exercise plan or alternative exercises like yoga, dance, or a health spa. We shall analyze for you what is good and what is lacking in all of these. Then it is up to you to use your own judgment, assessing your needs and your goals to decide if you wish to continue with your own life-style or combine it with our program.

We can guarantee to lead you into the best principles for exercise, demonstrate these principles in a coordinated basic series of multipurpose exercises to *maintain* your present body fitness (if you're satisfied with that), help you *attain* a better fitness level (if that is your goal), or serve as a fifteen-minute *warm-up* for a more strenuous program of physical activity. This basic series we call the Master Plan.

Now, the Master Plan is complete in itself. It links a set of unique exercises, devised by Miss Harrison, into a smooth progression from one starting position. Each series of exercises advances you from the easy-to-do to the more demanding. You control the pace; but as your body becomes more accustomed to its movement, you will be able to promote yourself and conquer the more difficult ones.

The Master Plan is realistic and definitive, because it stretches, warms up, and strengthens your muscles. In just about fifteen minutes, it activates all parts of your body and starts you on the important task of becoming limber and firming up.

For those of you who grow to love movement, the Master Plan becomes the foundation for a more developed exercise program. And it is an excellent warm-up for any sports activity.

Do you feel you don't need an entire Master Plan? We have some options for you (see page 58). Want to work on those areas where fat has accumulated and mars the general outline? ("Cellulite," if it makes you feel happier.) Use your Master Plan options, then check the table of contents for the areas you wish to work on. Select all of the exercises, or a few of the exercises, *but do the exercises you select faithfully.* Consistency is the key to recontouring your landscape.

However, you might be surprised about your physical-fitness needs. Before you decide on the bits-and-pieces approach to exercise, why not take the tests we have devised to provide you with a realistic picture of yourself and your personal needs? You can score your own "Movement Profile" to discover if you move, how you move, and if it is enough movement for you, the real physical you.

Many people have areas of their body that are "frozen." What we mean by this is, they feel uncomfortable and fail to utilize certain parts of their body.

Our studies showed, for example, that when we asked a client to move his rib cage, he was unaware that he was able to move it independently of other parts of his body. Does this apply to you? Why not check to see?

Do you have an awareness of your body in motion? Is it graceful, or do you consider yourself clumsy? We can show you how to move more freely by unlocking the frozen areas and limbering them up. As you become more supple and freer, the way you appear to others will change, and you will learn to be comfortable with your body and its movements.

The planned and creative use of movement therapy developed through the Movement Profile in Chapter 3 is a new key concept. The techniques you learn will enhance your life. Other chapters will show you how to exercise together as a family (for both physical and social benefits); how exercise can be sensuous and part of an increased enjoyment of sex; how exercise can alleviate back pain; and how to continue your exercises while working or traveling. There is also a special chapter on how to relax.

By now, you must have the idea that we believe exercise is important in your life and that adding it to your everyday activities will not only make you more attractive but also make you feel better.

We could underline the medical benefits again and again: the facts that you will lose weight more easily, that your circulation improves, that you lessen the risk of heart attack and cardiovascular disease—these are cold, scientific facts.

We know we are dealing with warm, human people. When you say you want to lose weight, you mean you want to look better.

Scientific or human, the exercise approach is the one to take. We promise we'll make it easy and fun. Read on. The rest is up to you!

2 Alternative Programs: The Perils of Fad Exercise

One question we are frequently asked is, "What about the miracles—the back-of-the-magazine ads for books and devices that promise an easy-off of extra inches? How about the gyms, spas, and exercise clubs? Do dance classes help? Should I study yoga?"

The woods are populated by people who are searching for the No-Exercise Exercise Program. It has not, as yet, been invented. However, in fairness to our readers, we feel that we must comment on some of the more prevalent forms of "no-exercise" or "alternative-exercise" programs.

Let's start with the gyms, spas, and exercise clubs. They are not necessarily interchangeable terms. To begin with, many spas are beauty shops in disguise. The exercise equipment is a front to lure in the person with extra time and cash. A great deal of consumer education has taken place in this field. All of it points to two suggestions: (1) Read over carefully any contract that you sign for long-term membership in a spa. (2) Investigate thoroughly beforehand the facilities and the training of the people involved.

Alternative Programs: Perils of Fad Exercise

See what kind of guidance you receive and if it individualizes the program for you. Think about any medical problem you may have that their equipment might aggravate.

Many offer pools, but a swimming pool is only as good as its size and upkeep. Obviously, the true swimmer will be a fish out of water in an indoor pool the size of one in a suburban Long Island spa—it is barely ten feet across in each direction. However, even a pool of such limited size can be used in an exercise program, because the extra energy required to move in the water increases the effectiveness of exercise. Decide what you want in the way of swimming; if the pool fits, then it might be worthwhile for you.

Quite frequently a more luxurious spa will offer a whirlpool, sauna, and steam room as a come-on. These are all luxurious for the tired and tense, but do not expect that they will ever take the place of exercise. They should be *carefully* used for relieving both mental and muscular tension. Heat may temporarily "sweat off" a few pounds, but it is an illusory loss, one that is dissipated with the first glass of water.

So that you will understand the type of exercise program if you are investigating a spa or gym, there are three terms that you must know. (1) *Isotonic Exercise:* This is exercise that involves simply moving a weight through the range of motion of a joint. (2) *Isokinetic:* This is exercise that adds a constant resistance through the range of motion of a joint. *Isometrics:* These are exercises that were popular several years ago which involve the tensing and contracting of muscles without actual physical movement. Their exclusive use has fallen into disfavor because they tend to develop bulky muscles and because they do not require energy enough to improve heart and lung action. Also, there is no control of the amount of force exerted on a joint.

There are gyms and there are gyms. Many offer fitness

equipment that works on an isokinetic principle. For some, this equipment, with very light weights, can be beneficial in tightening flabby muscles. Beware of the place that is equipped with hyperactive reducing machines where you are promised that *you* need not expend any energy at all. The machine may shake, quake, jiggle, and vibrate you. The machine may relax and soothe you or be upsettingly uncomfortable in its attack on your flesh. It will not, however, take off any weight or any inches.

True gyms, with equipment like bars, beams, and horses, require experts to teach and experts to use. They are excellent for all-around fitness programs, but the novice needs careful instruction in use and safety. If you are interested in a gym like this, be certain that your membership includes instruction in the use of all equipment. Be certain that there is an instructor on hand to observe while the equipment is in use. Above all, be sure that you have worked up to a program of vigorous exercise before you undertake participation in a fast game of basketball, handball, or volleyball. If your muscles have been sitting around relaxing for years, your entire body may rebel at a sudden reintroduction to strenuous activity.

The ultimate in no-exercise programs is the use of massage. Massage will not do anything to redistribute the accumulation of fat. Even when a massage has been vigorous enough to cause black-and-blue marks, the fat deposit will not be broken up. Nor does massage have any effect on the muscle tone.

Massage *can* be beneficial, for example, when you have muscles that are fatigued. A good massage will increase circulation to an area and help you feel better. After serious injury, massage can help maintain muscles in a state of better nutrition until a program of rehabilitation can be begun.

The final offering of the gym or spa is generally an exer-

Alternative Programs: Perils of Fad Exercise

cise class. This is where investigation is especially necessary. Two years ago there was an article published which exposed the behind-the-scenes of one of the largest chains of spas. It was written by a woman who had had no training at all in exercising but had been hired because she was thin and graceful. The article detailed her experiences, including an incident where she had to call an ambulance for a man who had passed out while exercising on the isokinetic machines. No one present had had sufficient training to recognize that the man was in physical distress. This is precisely what you don't want in the line of an exercise instructor. Perhaps your best warning flag is a sales pitch that promises that you will lose ten pounds in seven days. When you hear a promise like that, beware! The ethics of the establishment can well be suspect.

Perhaps one of the most popular "alternative exercises" is dance. Classes in all types of dance, from folk and ballroom through belly, are offered on the grounds that the exercise is good for the participant. Folk or ballroom dancing for an evening may be an attractive activity for those who might never move a muscle otherwise.

Modern dance is an excellent way to exercise. But sometimes the warm-up exercises for these groups frequently involve a bobbing technique that could put too much stress on untrained muscles. If this is the sort of exercise attractive to you, seek out an "eclectic" teacher who designs her classes to suit the needs of her students.

As for belly dancing, it is a fad of the moment that is fast fading. What it has going for it is that it is so frequently advertised as the "sexy way to exercise." With jangle belt and finger cymbals, to say nothing of navel jewel, thousands of women are being lured into exercise sessions. If it intrigues you, fine. Just remember that very few belly dancers possess flat bellies. Also, the deeply arched positions can put excessive stress on the lower back. If you have back or joint problems of any kind, belly dancing is not for you.

Another of the more exotic types of exercise often resorted to is yoga. Yoga, it should be remembered, is really a system of Indian religious philosophy that stresses unity of human spirit and universal spirit. The postures (asanas) required of the yoga student should discipline the mind and create a strong, healthy body through developing flexibility of joints and spinal column. There are benefits to heart and lungs to be achieved by controlling the abdominal breathing. However, the energy output is minimal, and general endurance does not grow from the use of yoga. In addition, many of the positions advocated are not comfortable for women, for the very good reason that in India the yogis were men. The arched-back positions do what belly dancing does—they put excessive stress on the lower back. Also, certain positions in yoga can aggravate an existing neck or back problem.

Our stand on yoga is that it serves as an introduction to body movement that is beneficial for some. Others may find it not only boring but also painful. The yoga claim to assistance in weight control must be balanced against the awareness that yogis not only practice yoga but also practice fasting and subsist on a Spartan diet.

What about the books that are published with such great regularity? The first great category consists of what we think of as "body-beautiful books." The largest splash lately among these has been made by the books on cellulite. These books all pander to the female proclivity to put on fat in the characteristic pattern of padding on the hips, thighs, buttocks, abdomen, and arms. The thesis of the books is that this fat is *special*, that it differs from other types of fat. The books claim that it can be attacked by tranquil thoughts, a diet, and eight glasses of water daily. Readers

Alternative Programs: Perils of Fad Exercise 29

are encouraged to stroke and massage away the pads of fat—*spot reduction,* by any other term. Again, the unproved thesis (by medical standards) put forth by many cellulite authors is that this fat is different. There are no such things as "polluting" and "nonpolluting" foods, and eight glasses of water a day could harm someone with a kidney problem. The books appeal because they speak so directly to the problem that bedevils even women who may not be overweight in terms of the weight charts. However, these plans do not offer anything that will alleviate the problem that is not better done by a sincere program of exercise and a nutritionally balanced diet. The best thing that can be said about the most popular of these books is that the pictures are pretty.

More exercises may be found in the second category of books that we loosely think of as the "physical-fitness books" because they are more directly related to body tone than body appearance. Among the first of these books were the *RCAF XBS Plan for Women* and the *RCAF 5BX Plan for Men.* These books offer a series of exercises with graduated difficulty. Each set of exercises is to be followed until a specified number of repetitions are accomplished within a certain amount of time. The repetitions are increased within the time span until a maximum level is reached. At that point a new series of exercises is begun. Variations within the series are allowed according to age, and each exerciser adjusts the program to her or his own rate of progress. The basic flaw in this plan is that not *all* muscle groups are exercised in each series.

Dr. Kenneth Cooper, a respected exercise cardiologist, is responsible for a book titled *Aerobics* and for a whole school of exercising that has grown from it. Basically the term refers to exercises that stimulate heart and lung activity long enough to have a beneficial physiological effect.

His exercises for women include walking, running, cycling, swimming, stair climbing, and rope skipping. Depending on the individual program selected, progress is made by going farther, and faster, determining by heart checks at what point the next level of exercise should be begun. Although the critics say the program does not place any emphasis on strength or flexibility, in fairness to Dr. Cooper, it was not planned to do that. Distance and duration determine progress, and heart checks are used to monitor this.

Currently the book that is most quoted is Dr. Laurence Morehouse's *Total Fitness in 30 Minutes a Week*. This combines calisthenics and aerobic activity to achieve a certain heart rate for a specified period. The title is misleading, for it refers only to the thirty minutes during the week that are allotted in ten-minute periods to develop a "reserve of fitness." These include one minute of limbering exercise, four minutes of muscle building (push-ups and partial sit-backs), plus five minutes of activity to lift the heart rate to the desired level (a variety of running-in-place activity). Moreover, Dr. Morehouse completes his program by including the daily turning and twisting of the joints, standing for two hours every day, carrying a weight for five seconds per day, raising the heart rate to 120 beats for at least three minutes, and burning up 300 calories in physical activity. The latter, for a woman, could be accomplished by walking briskly for one hour per day. All this is in addition to the basic thirty minutes per week of the title!

The Official YMCA Physical Fitness Handbook contains an exercise plan that is ostensibly for both men and women. While these exercises are properly graduated from warm-up through cool-off and include a postgraduate course, the stress on arm and leg strength is more suited to men than women.

What about sports as a form of exercise?

Alternative Programs: Perils of Fad Exercise

This is a qualified "yes." It would be an unqualified "yes" if only people maintained an interest in their favorite sport throughout their adult lives. Too many, however, are enthusiastic participants during their late teens and early twenties, and only sometime participants as they arrive in their thirties. Suddenly the forties and fifties arrive, accompanied by the forty and fifty waistlines. Immediately the ex-tennis buff, the onetime golfer, and the aging swimmer decide to return to their fields of glory.

This is dangerous. Such returns should be gradual. A program of progressively strengthening exercises to tone muscles and revive heart and lung capacity needs to be instituted. At the very least, the returnee should limit the amount of participation at the outset, and gradually build to a *reasonable* participation for his age and physical condition. Again, there is no one better qualified to advise on this than the family doctor or heart specialist.

The range of sports for adults is generally restricted from B through W. When patients discuss sports with me, I find that the definition is limited to: "How about bowling, golf, swimming, tennis, or walking-jogging?" There are very few other physical activities generally accepted by the adult populace, so let's address ourselves to what you can expect from regular indulgence in one of these five—all of which are basically throwing movements, running movements, or a combination of both.

Bowling contributes the least in the way of pure exercise, requiring neither strength nor endurance. But it does build rhythm and coordination. It is also relaxing and gives many people a chance to socialize. Give this exercise good marks for recreation and relaxation.

Golf is a many-things-to-many-people game. The effect it has on your physical fitness is totally up to you. You can play it the hard way—carrying your clubs and walking briskly around the course, thereby increasing slightly the effect the game has on your respiratory system. Or you can dog it in a golf cart, hopping off your vehicle for a leisurely swing at the inoffensive ball, and continuing on around the eighteen holes in this fashion. Obviously, you don't obtain much real exercise from pressing your foot against the accelerator. You might find the twisting of the swing good for the waistline, but it still does not qualify as a real physical-fitness activity. Golf for exercise is just like a washing machine—you'll get out of it exactly what you put in.

Swimming enthusiasts insist that theirs is the complete exercise. Research by Dr. Thomas K. Cureton, professor of physical education, University of Illinois, bears the enthusiasts out. Regular swimming, as shown in Cureton's study, lowers the pulse rate, improves lung capacity and cardiovascular capacity (for the asthmatic, this is a real benefit), increases breath-holding ability, strengthens the legs and arms, builds endurance, and reduces body fat. With all that going for it, you know there has to be a qualifying element. There is. You must swim *regularly* to obtain these benefits. Daily immersion is best, but popping into the pool or the ocean two or three times a week will give you a lot of results for the time spent. You must swim—not fanny-dip or float. Moving against the resistance of the water is what counts in swimming. Swimming is excellent for people with weight-bearing joint problems. It can take an arthritic joint through a normal range of motion without the stress of weight bearing, and therefore help maintain flexibility and muscle strength, which in turn help relieve stress and pain in the joints.

As for tennis, its effect on your cardiorespiratory system depends on how vigorous you are and how often you play. Naturally, the more sustained, the better the effects,

Alternative Programs: Perils of Fad Exercise

except that, again, the good results come with a very important warning. If you are over thirty, this game could be dangerous if you have not played regularly in a long period of time. Tennis is a game of agility, concentration, endurance, and quickness. When you condition for tennis, you'll want to work on suppleness and strength. Whether you play doubles or singles, your stroke is important. Your arm and shoulder have to be strong enough to give power to your game, and your legs have to be tough and tireless.

The final category in the heading of "sports" is walking-jogging. Let's begin with a definition. By walking-jogging, what I mean medically is the sort of walking-jogging that is included in the aerobic exercises—it stimulates heart and lung activity long enough to have a beneficial effect, and it is done at a brisk pace. Even at that, it takes three miles of activity to burn up 250 calories. In practical terms, you'll walk three miles a day for two weeks to lose a pound. If that sounds discouraging, consider that losing 36 pounds of fat every year is no mean accomplishment. What's more, you are walking for more than weight loss; you are walking for physical fitness.

We encourage my patients and Evalee's clients to walk as much as possible, because both of us believe that it is one of the best exercises for all ages. Our exercise plan endorses movement, so we endorse walking in addition to the plan. The leisurely stroll is out: you'll know you are walking when you are clipping along at a pace of about four miles per hour. This will really provide you with worthwhile fitness benefits.

Jogging is actually walking done a little faster, or running slowed down. Obviously, the brisker the pace, the better the results from a standpoint of fitness. Many medical authorities feel that jogging on a regular basis improves the function of the heart, blood vessels, and lungs. It can certainly increase the amount of oxygen carried to the tissues of the body.

What happens is this. Additional blood vessels are formed in skeletal and heart muscles as a result of the demands on the body while jogging or running. (This is one of the unpaid side benefits that professional athletes enjoy as a result of their professions.) Developing this collateral blood-vessel system is like money in the bank for your body. With the process of aging, when your original supply of blood vessels begins to give way to wear and tear, you have another system to take over part of the load. Should the main vessel supplying the heart be clogged by cholesterol, the secondary system will keep the heart from dying by carrying oxygen to it. Why not jog along and live longer?

Just remember before starting a jogging program that you should get the okay from your doctor that your heart is sound and you are fit enough. You should begin slowly and work up the pace gradually, ideally under some knowledgeable supervision.

Only your doctor can tailor-make an *optimum* exercise program for you, and you should consult him before you start—not on the way to the Emergency Room. It is with certain reservations that we insert the following information, but it does belong. It is not meant to frighten or alarm. The purpose is to give you all the facts. If at any time when you are exercising you experience chest pain that does or does not run down one or both arms, stop! Immediately rest and notify your doctor. Many people who received their first intimation of heart trouble in this way are alive today because they heeded the warning of this type of pain. Those who fail to listen to what their hearts were telling them are those who make the obituary pages and whose friends say, "But he was always the picture of health!"

I do not feel that slowly building physical skills will expose anyone to this danger. What I intend by the warning is to have you begin slowly and sensibly and not rush in to take on Billie Jean King for your first tennis match.

The natural place for women to seek some exercise guidance would seem to be the weight-control groups that are flourishing. Among those that are national in scope, only the Diet Workshop offers exercise as part of its regular weight-reduction program. Until this year, Diet Workshop members have been taught simple isotonic exercises designed to be done while sitting in a chair, fully clothed. These activities were planned to tone the body during the period of weight loss. At the same time, the instructors within the groups encourage members to undertake physical activity as a means of burning up calories more efficiently. At present, the Diet Workshop is planning a new program called Body Design. These exercises will be for instructors and members who are on maintenance, and they are based on the exercises to be found in this book.

Now you know about alternative exercise programs. Are they for you? You have the facts; the decision is yours. The purpose has been to give you the information so that you may intelligently decide, not *if* you will exercise, but *how* you will exercise.

3 All About You: Defining Your Own Needs

Did you know that you have a Movement Profile, and it's a part of you all the time? It's how you enter a room, how you sit and stand. It is the "moving you."

There are two specific aspects to your Movement Profile. First, there's your "expressive style" of movement that is uniquely yours. This quality is reflected in the way you use your body and the space around you. It's how you move with, toward, and away from others.

Second, there is your "activity style." This includes the various kinds of physical exertion that you engage in daily, and the subsequent calories you burn up as a result. For example, a secretary's caloric expenditure is normally much less than that of a woman on the move all day with three small children.

So, then, expressive style plus activity style equals your Movement Profile. The really wonderful thing about your Movement Profile is that it is changeable. If your activity

All About You: Defining Your Own Needs

style has placed parts of your body in the deep-freeze, this will affect your expressive style. You cannot move gracefully when some of your joints are nearly immovable.

Where are you now? And what do you need to change? Two simple tests can reveal a person's Movement Profile. The first determines your expressive style by revealing which parts of your body, if any, are "frozen." The second determines your activity style. What you learn gives you the insight to change. Here are the tests that we ask you to try. We think that you will be encouraged and interested by the results. Test #1 has eight simple parts.

TEST 1. YOUR EXPRESSIVE STYLE: How to Pinpoint Frozen Body Areas

You may not be aware of the areas of your body that have fallen into disuse and become stiff and unyielding. Try the following eight exercises to discover just where you are frozen into place. You'll be amazed at the instant feedback that you get from your body. All you need is a ball, or balloon, about eight inches in diameter.

DIRECTIONS: Try each exercise twice, and move only that part of the body described. Try to eliminate any other motion. If available, use a mirror to check your movements. When an exercise is easy to perform, try to increase your range of movement by holding the ball farther away from your body, or stand farther from the wall, etc.

POSITION 1: Stand with legs hip-width apart and knees slightly bent. Hold ball with both hands approximately two inches in front of pelvis.

MOVEMENT: Without bending at the waist, try to swing your pelvis forward until the ball is touched. Swing your pelvis back to center position after each try. If the ball is easily touched, try to increase your range of movement by increasing the distance of the ball by one inch. *Note:* To unfreeze this area, isolate this movement by not moving any other parts of your body.

POSITION 2: Same as Position 1. Hold the ball two inches behind buttocks with both hands.

MOVEMENT: Swing your pelvis back until ball is touched. Return to center. The rest of the body remains in place. If the ball is easily touched, try to increase your range of movement by increasing the distance one inch farther from body.

All About You: Defining Your Own Needs

POSITION 3: Same as Position 1. Hold the ball with both hands two inches from your chest.

MOVEMENT: Without moving your lower body, or bending from the waist, try to push your chest and rib-cage area forward until the ball is touched. Return to center position.

POSITION 4: Stand with right side to the wall, feet parallel, hip-width apart, and knees slightly bent. Measure eight inches from the wall to the inside of your right foot. Clasp your hands in front of your body.

MOVEMENT: Swing your hips over until the right hip touches wall. Hold one count. Swing your hips back to center. Do not tilt your upper body. Stand with left side to wall and repeat exercise.

POSITION 5: Stand. Place hands on hips and grip them firmly.

MOVEMENT: Slowly roll your shoulders forward, up, back, and down in a continuous circular motion. After one circle, reverse direction. Move only your shoulders.

POSITION 6: Stand relaxed.

MOVEMENT: Slowly draw in your abdominal muscles. Hold for three counts. Release slowly. Repeat abdominal contractions three times without tensing up other parts of your body or holding your breath.

POSITION 7: Stand relaxed.

MOVEMENT: Slowly pull in and tighten your buttock muscles. Hold for a count of three. Release slowly. Try to tighten your right buttock. Hold for two counts and release. Tighten your left buttock, hold for two counts, and release. During tensing, keep other parts of your body relaxed and your breathing even and natural.

POSITION 8: Stand relaxed.

MOVEMENT: Slowly turn your head until your chin is over your left shoulder. Hold. Use your nose as a pen, and, moving from left to right shoul-

All About You: Defining Your Own Needs   41

der, write or print your full name in space. After your name is written, move from right to left to erase it with your chin.

This is one test in which hardly anyone scores 100 percent, so don't be discouraged. Most people experience some difficulty. Ninety-one out of one hundred patients in my medical study were like you. They discovered that parts of their upper or lower bodies were frozen. Of course, they didn't like this discovery, and perhaps you share some of their feelings in these comments.

Mrs. J. said, "I feel disconnected from my lower body. Of course, I know it is there, but I feel I am just dragging it around."

Mr. P. added this comment: "I jog a lot, and when I'm jogging, I am aware that my shoulders feel like a deadweight. I'd like to free them up, but I don't know how."

"I discovered that I had no freedom in my pelvis. It isn't loose at all. In fact, it feels like a wooden board," was Miss L.'s contribution.

Mr. H. came up with this observation: "My rib cage is a complete blank to me. I have never used this area of my body, and I have never been aware of its moving for any purpose at all."

Another revealing remark came from Mrs. C., who claimed, "When I walk, I feel my buttocks are hanging there like a deadweight, pulling me backward and off balance, and I feel awkward."

What I discovered to be significant for my patients was that weight didn't seem to be the determining factor for the frozen body areas. Over half the people I tested characterized themselves as being an ideal weight, but they still felt that they had uncomfortable body areas that they could not move freely enough. Thawing these uncomfortable areas is one reason for an exercise program.

The old adage "You are what you eat" could be easily changed to "You are how you move." Your body is going to reflect what portions of it you move during the day and the conditions under which you move it. Assembly-line workers who stand in one spot and move only a small set of muscles will have to work hard to have the overall agility of O. J. Simpson or Chrissie Evert. Dull, repetitive movement; tense, stressful situations; lack of exercise—all contribute to your physical form and your mental attitude.

The next test we have for you is mental rather than physical. It is a series of self-accountability questions. The plain, straightforward truth will assist you to an overview of how you spend your time physically. Again, the goal is insight—insight that will help you change your patterns and habits if they do not fit into the activity style you would like to project.

TEST 2. YOUR ACTIVITY AWARENESS

DIRECTIONS: Answer each question with yes or no.

_____ Are you breathless after climbing a flight of stairs?
_____ Are most of your physical activities relegated to weekends?
_____ Are you often physically tired even though you have not been engaged in any strenuous activity?
_____ Are your hobbies or recreation and entertainment mostly passive and spectator type rather than active and physically involved? (Theater, concerts, TV

All About You: Defining Your Own Needs 43

viewing vs. hiking, camping, bowling, folk dancing.)
_____ Does sporadic physical activity leave you feeling stiff and out of shape?
_____ Do you often use your car to run errands even when they are within walking distance?
Does your activity fall into
_____ light,
_____ moderate,
_____ heavy energy expenditure?
_____ Do you expend yourself physically every day in walking, gardening, shopping, or household chores?
Are you most active physically
_____ in the morning,
_____ afternoon,
_____ evening?
_____ Do you use your phone or secretary for communication within the office or work place when you could walk instead?

Are you surprised by how limited your awareness really is? Do you see some areas where you could be more active?

If you are now interested in increasing your energy output, the next step is to review a typical day in your life. Think about your average day in relation to the amount of energy you put into it. You have undoubtedly developed some patterns that ease you through the hours. You've discovered how to cut a few steps here, save a little energy there, sit a little longer, and stand a little less. Now you must undo this mode of thinking and go into reverse. Back up across your acquired patterns to uncover the simple ways in which you may start to burn more calories by putting more movement in your life. Here is the basic list I recommend:

Stand rather than sit every time you can.

Park your car farther away from work, school, store, or errands. Then walk briskly to your destination. Best place to park the car when possible? At home!

Get off the bus at least two stops from your destination and walk a few extra blocks.

At work, deliver messages and memos personally rather than picking up the phone or using the intercom.

Use the stairs to a lavatory one flight up or down.

Avoid elevators. If your office is in a high-rise building, get off and walk the last three flights.

Plan five active minutes every evening—walk the dog, mail a letter, run an errand.

Start the morning and the day with activity before you get out of bed by devising a simple warm-up stretching routine for daily use.

I have had great feedback from my own patients. Once you place a body in motion, it tends to remain in motion—that's a basic law of physics. My placed-in-motion patients have enthusiastically endorsed these as ways of staying in motion:

Running or jogging in place during television commercials. (Notice, I said in place—not to the refrigerator.)

Joining a hiking, biking, jogging, or sport group.

Forming an exercise group within your own apartment building, neighborhood, or office. Alternate leadership in each other's homes to keep it interesting. Use the exercises in this book, but choose ones appealing to everyone.

Take a movement class in something you have never tried before: tap dancing, primitive dancing, jazz dancing, tai chi, karate, etc.

All About You: Defining Your Own Needs

Make up a list of "short-term" errands or activities possible during the week. Choose one per day. Update the list weekly with activities that require effort on your part. Volunteer to teach or assist with a movement or activity class in a school, senior-citizen home, nursery, etc.

You've just been involved with identifying your own problem areas. You have seen how these can affect your life-style. I have offered you some options for change from my own suggestions and from suggestions of people just like you. You can do something about it; but before you begin, you must prepare. Insulting your unused muscles with sudden overwhelming demands may send those poor muscles into spasm. Are you ready to begin?

Part II

4 Priming for Exercise

How can anything so good for you as exercise turn so many people off? Many have been discouraged by routines that are dull, unrealistic, or too strenuous. Coaxing your figure to stay in line is no fun if you have to coax yourself constantly to do something you don't enjoy. Evalee and I have found that what works best is a program that leads you onward, encouraging you to expand your activities. Those who have tried it say that our *stem-progression technique* fills this need because the continuity of movement, gradual buildup, and variety of exercise keep them constantly interested.

UNDERSTANDING THE TERMS

Like anything that is unique, our exercise program has its own vocabulary. To avoid misunderstanding between us, we are taking the time to make the definitions before you begin. (The Glossary in the back of this book will also prove useful.) Once you have read through your vocabulary list, you'll see more clearly where you are headed and how to get there with exercises that are fun to do.

STEM-PROGRESSION TECHNIQUE

Each series of exercises begins with a *"stem position"*—the basic position with exact directions for precise placement of hand, arms, trunk, and legs. The subsequent exercises for the set originate from the pictured stem. (This holds true for the exercises for areas of concentration where you trim down fatty deposits—*cellulite,* in various parts of the body.)

The exercises progress in order of difficulty from the easiest, to the intermediate, to the advanced and hardest to execute. In each group, the last exercise is the most demanding. You will discover that the variations flow naturally from one to the other, because each is an extension of the previous one. This progression leads to linking the exercises in a series that may be completed without breaking the rhythm or the continuity.

You'll find that although the exercise pattern for each area of the body remains the same, with each step there is an increasing demand upon specific muscles, or that you will be working a different set of muscles within each area of concentration. This will make you more and more aware of your body.

Each exercise chapter contains several stem positions. These become your monitoring devices. As your capacity to exercise develops, you will note it by your ability to move on to the next movement in the stem. It's a sure sign your body is shaping up and that you are ready to graduate to the next level.

LATERAL TORSO BENDING

When our long-ago ancestors decided to stand on two feet, they unwittingly made us heirs to many problems. One of these problems is the amount of stress we place on our side muscles, muscles that must work constantly under tension to keep us upright. Movements to the side relax these muscles, so when the trunk is to be exercised, it is imperative to begin with a side-bending movement *before* bending forward. By doing this, you allow one set of muscles to relax while the other is contracting.

QUALITY

The consistency and rhythm of your exercises contributes to quality. When you rush through the program, you are cheating yourself of the quality. Smooth and unhurried movements, begun slowly, are important. Once you have moved to one side, move to the other an equal number of times. Always give your body time to adjust to increasing demands on it.

BODY STABILIZATION

Your body should be placed in the exact position for every exercise. Make only the movements prescribed; don't add any of your own. When your body is locked into position for the prescribed motions, those motions have more impact because resistance among the muscle groups increases demands on other muscles and gives you the maximum benefit from the exercise.

SAFETY

As a medical man, I feel these exercises are safe for all ages, provided you have no precluding medical problem. As a doctor, I must also add yet again that before you embark on this, *or on any other exercise program,* you should consult your own physician.

That warning is most important. You may have some hidden problem that makes modification of the program necessary in your case, and your doctor is the one who will know this. His advice takes precedence.

TAPERING OFF

Just as you begin slowly and warm up, you should end gradually and cool off. After each session of exercise, walk around at a moderate pace, shaking your wrists. Help your heart to slow down to its normal beat by breathing slowly and deeply in through your nose and out through your mouth for about three minutes.

Here is an interesting fact to remember. Drinking cold beverages immediately after exercise can be dangerous, because the cold liquid going down the esophagus passes directly in front of the heart. In a *few* susceptible people, this icy shock could even stop the heart.

GUIDELINES

Now that you understand the basic glossary of exercise terms, there are a few general guidelines to follow as you proceed through the exercises that have been devised for you and your body trimming.

1. If you have eaten a large meal, wait for thirty min-

utes before you begin to exercise. That way you decrease the chance of nausea.

2. You should drink at least a quart of fluid daily. Your own thirst will give you the best guide to the amount that you require. However, I have discovered that people new to exercising do not realize that they need to replace the fluid lost through physical exertion, and they become dehydrated. These are the people who complain that they feel tired and irritable from exercise, when all they need is some fluid intake. Immediately after replacing the lost fluid, they replace their irritability and fatigue with a sense of invigoration and relaxation.

3. Wear the proper clothing for exercising. Notice, I said proper, not special. Shorts or slacks with a T-shirt allow freedom of motion. Bare feet are fine for any exercise not performed standing, and even then if the exercise is specifically for the muscles of the feet. Otherwise, wear sneakers or some other comfortable flat-cushioned shoes.

4. Give yourself the luxury of time. Put aside fifteen uninterrupted minutes out of the day and use this fifteen minutes to do as many of the exercises as possible. When you are unaccustomed to exercising, you may want to extend this time period, because it does take longer to perform when you are not so familiar with what you are doing. You will discover that you can go through the Master Plan faster and become increasingly expert each time you do it.

5. Be regular in exercising. Once a day is best for the Master Plan. Three times a week is adequate. Twice a week is minimum. Think of it this way: Aren't you important

enough in your life to deserve a small segment of time each day to keep yourself healthier?

6. If the number of times stated for an exercise is too much, reduce it to a number comfortable for you and increase as endurance permits. The reason we have so many repetitions for each exercise is to guarantee you improved fitness and increased circulatory benefits. You may reach your goal more slowly, depending on your present level of fitness.

7. Be sure that you have something soft between you and the floor. A mat or a carpet will ward off the damp and the bruises. Never exercise directly on concrete, but a wooden floor won't hurt you in floor exercises.

8. Have fun. Play the sort of music you like, and exercise in time to the beat. Anything that is bright and peppy makes a good background for physical movement and energizes you to keep going.

Now that you have the background, it is time to begin.

5 The Master Plan

The Master Plan is an exercise program that is multipurpose. Depending on the level you seek, the Master Plan serves you in the following ways: to *attain* basic physical fitness; as a *warm-up* to be used prior to further exercise, or if already fit; as a maintenance program.

The Master Plan is a total-body approach. It will increase your awareness of your body, increase your fitness, and help you maintain your new appearance while making you feel truly alive. All this is enough, but you will look better, too.

We have organized the Master Plan so that it is easy to follow. You work from the head down to the toes by starting with head and neck movements, then putting each section of the body into action.

There is no guesswork in the Master Plan. The directions are explicit. The advisable minimum as well as the maximum goals are set out. Because of the stem-progression technique, you will find each series of exercises easy to do and easy to remember. You will be adding new movements almost daily, so the program varies constantly.

Pace your exercising to your own particular tempo and temperament. We advise you to start slowly and work first only on the exercises that you can do without too much strain or difficulty. Once you have familiarized yourself with the Master Plan, you should be able to complete it easily within fifteen minutes.

You are nearly ready to begin working on the Master Plan. Before you do, I have a few more last-minute reminders, the same ones that I go over with my patients when I work with them personally. If you were in my office, this is what I would tell you to do.

1. If you are using the Master Plan to *attain* fitness or simply for a warm-up exercise, use the minimum number of times stated.

2. Always start with Stem 1, Movement A. Do Movement A the minimum number of times. Your goal is to work up to the maximum. Stop at any point in Stem 1 when the movements become too difficult to do and proceed to Stem 2, Movement A, for the minimum number. Again, stop at the point in Stem 2 when the movements become too difficult, and go on to Stem 3. Each day you should find that you are able to add a few movements to your repertoire. Do not force yourself to do movements your muscles are not prepared to do. Your body will let you know when it is free enough to undertake more demands.

3. Your goal, if using the Master Plan solely for maintenance, should be to work gradually up to the *maximum* number of exercises and to do these in fifteen minutes. How long it takes you to reach this point depends on your physical state when you begin your exercise program. It is completely different for everyone who tries it. If you

are using the Master Plan to *attain* fitness or simply for a warm-up exercise, use the minimum number of times stated.

4. Exercises 1–4 are completed from a floor position. To avoid foot cramp during the seated portion of an exercise, you may change your leg positions to any of the following as you need: tailor fashion, with legs crossed at ankles; diamond pattern, with soles and heels pressed together and knees out to the side; or hip-flexed, with knees together and bent and feet resting flat on the floor.

5. Always stretch your body to each side before stretching forward. This will allow your back muscles to relax properly.

6. Caution: begin each set of exercises slowly, but do speed up the pace and exert more effort as soon as you can. You will see results faster when you do.

7. Whenever the term "hold" is used, keep the position for one count. You should be maintaining a steady beat as you exercise.

8. At the end of every variation, return to the stem position.

9. Never hold your breath as you exercise.

10. It is imperative to cool off after going through the Master Plan or *any* strenuous exercise. Walk around, taking slow, deep breaths until you feel that your heartbeat has returned to normal.

11. Very important! Warning signs! Stop exercising if you:

> . . . become nauseated
> . . . start to tremble
> . . . experience any pain, particularly in the chest region
> . . . feel excessively fatigued
> . . . experience extreme weakness

58   DOCTOR SOLOMON

. . . notice excess perspiration
. . . become extremely flushed in the face
. . . notice heavy, labored breathing
. . . are suddenly overcome by dizziness

For those days when your time is short, we have provided you with a MASTER PLAN OPTION as follows: *If your goal is only to reduce one specific part of your body, we suggest you use Movement A of every Stem Position in the Master Plan before proceeding to exercises for specific parts. This guarantees that every part of your body gets properly warmed up.*

One final reminder: The Glossary in the back of the book will clarify any terms you are unsure about.

Now, for the Master Plan itself.

MASTER PLAN

AREA: Neck—Shoulders—Arms

STEM POSITION 1: ✓ Sit on floor. Legs crossed at ankles tailor fashion, or soles and heels pressed together, or feet on floor, knees bent. Body erect, weight slightly forward off the buttocks. Arms rest loosely over knees.

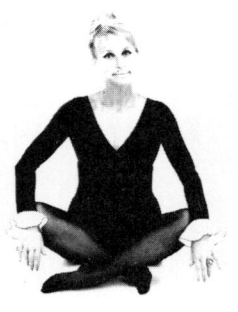

MOVEMENT A: ✓ Slowly turn head to right side until chin is over right shoulder. Hold. Return head to center.

The Master Plan

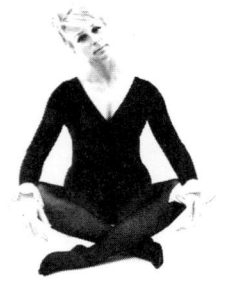

Hold. Slowly turn head until chin is over left shoulder. Hold. Return to center. Drop head forward, chin to chest. Hold. Lift head to center. Hold. Drop head back, chin to ceiling, jaw relaxed. Hold. Return to center. Incline head to right side by tilting ear to shoulder. Hold. Lift head to center. Hold. Incline head to left shoulder. Hold. Return to center. Hold. Extend head far forward. Hold. Pull head back. Hold.

TO ATTAIN FITNESS
OR FOR WARM-UP: Repeat series three times.

AS MAINTENANCE: Gradually work up to six.

MOVEMENT B: Slowly raise both shoulders up toward ears. Hold. Release and press shoulders down. Hold. Roll shoulders far forward. Hold. Press shoulders back. Hold.

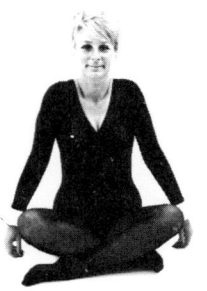

TO ATTAIN FITNESS
OR FOR WARM-UP: Repeat series four times.

AS MAINTENANCE: Gradually work up to eight times.

DOCTOR SOLOMON

MOVEMENT C: ✓

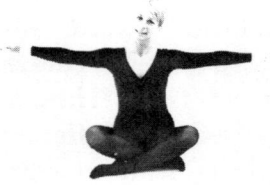

Make fists. Extend arms straight out from sides, shoulder level. Rotate arms forward in *big* circles eight times. Stop. Rotate arms back in *tight* circles eight times. Stop.

TO ATTAIN FITNESS
OR FOR WARM-UP: Repeat series three times.

AS MAINTENANCE: Gradually work up to six.

MOVEMENT D: Bend and cross arms in front around torso. Hold. Uncross, straighten, and swing arms to sides, shoulder level. Hold. Re-cross arms around torso. Hold. Uncross and swing to sides.

TO ATTAIN FITNESS
OR FOR WARM-UP: Repeat sequence ten times.

AS MAINTENANCE: Gradually work up to thirty.

MOVEMENT E: ✓

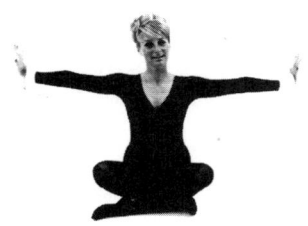

Extend arms out to sides, shoulder level, palms facing out, fingers up toward ceiling. Lift arms up overhead. Hold. Lower arms directly to the front, shoulder level. Hold. Lift arms overhead. Hold. Lower out to the sides.

TO ATTAIN FITNESS
OR FOR WARM-UP: Repeat sequence eight times.

AS MAINTENANCE: Gradually work up to twenty.

AREA: Waist—Midriff

STEM POSITION 2: Sit on floor. Feet pressed together. Knees open to sides. Arms loosely at sides.

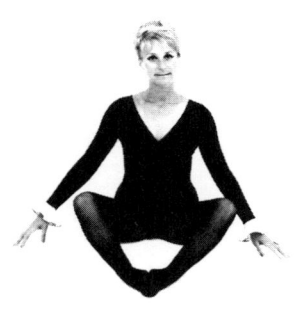

MOVEMENT A:

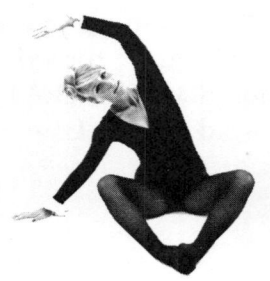

Place right hand to right side on floor. Curve left arm over head, palm up. Slowly bend to right side, right elbow bending to absorb deep bounce. Bounce toward floor four times before returning to upright position. Repeat movement to other side four times.

TO ATTAIN FITNESS OR FOR WARM-UP: Repeat groups of bounces four times to each side.

AS MAINTENANCE: Gradually work up to eight times on each side.

MOVEMENT B:

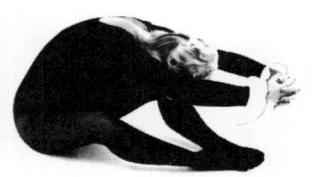

Bend forward from hips. Clasp hands. Stretch arms forward, head between arms. Slowly bounce forward and low over the floor four times. Slowly release torso upright with arms overhead.

TO ATTAIN FITNESS OR FOR WARM-UP: Repeat forward bounces four times.

AS MAINTENANCE: Gradually work up to eight times.

The Master Plan   63

MOVEMENT C: Place both hands on shoulders. Stretch right arm up straight overhead toward ceiling. As right arm lowers to shoulder, raise left arm straight overhead. Continue to alternate arms and strive to stretch upward as high as possible. Keep head slightly tilted back, and focus eyes to ceiling. With each reach, imagine lifting your waist up off your hips.

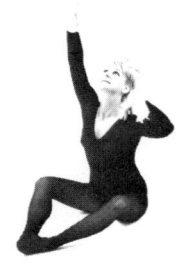

TO ATTAIN FITNESS
OR FOR WARM-UP: Repeat sequence ten times.

AS MAINTENANCE: Gradually work up to thirty times.

AREA: Legs—Feet—Ankles

STEM POSITION 3:   Sit on floor. Legs extended front. Toes pointed. Knees down. Arms relaxed at sides.

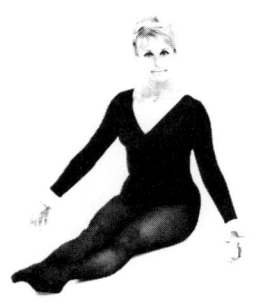

64 DOCTOR SOLOMON

MOVEMENT A:

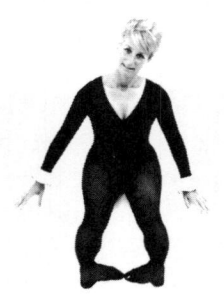

Turn feet toward each other until toes touch. Hold. Turn feet away from each other, toes outward as far as possible. Hold. Return feet to center. Point toes upward until heels flex. Hold. Point toes down. Hold. Release toes to center.

TO ATTAIN FITNESS
OR FOR WARM-UP: Repeat sequence four times.

AS MAINTENANCE: Gradually work up to ten times.

MOVEMENT B:

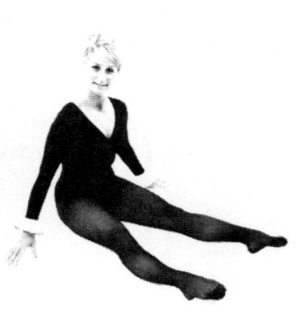

Slowly make circles with feet. Keep heels on floor. After four circles in one direction, reverse circles in opposite direction four times.

TO ATTAIN FITNESS
OR FOR WARM-UP: Repeat sequence four times on each side.

AS MAINTENANCE: Gradually work up to eight sets of circles.

The Master Plan 65

MOVEMENT C:

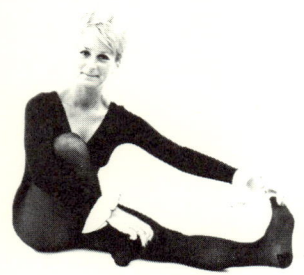

Flex feet. Point toes up. Bend knees and pull them to chest, heels on floor. Press knees together. Grasp toes with hands. Slide right leg forward on floor, as far as possible. Hold. Return knee to chest. Slide left leg forward on floor. Hold. Return knee to chest.

TO ATTAIN FITNESS OR FOR WARM-UP: Alternate legs and stretch six times.

AS MAINTENANCE: Gradually work up to twelve times.

STEM POSITION 4:

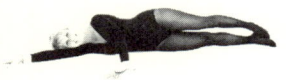

Lie on right side. Head resting on shoulder and arm. Left hand flat on floor by chest for support. Legs straight.

MOVEMENT A:

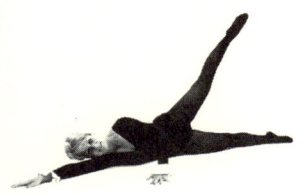

Raise left leg high off floor, toes pointed. Hold. Lower leg to stem position. Repeat on other side.

DOCTOR SOLOMON

TO ATTAIN FITNESS
OR FOR WARM-UP: Ten on each side.

AS MAINTENANCE: Twenty on each side.

MOVEMENT B: Raise left arm overhead until touching right hand. Simultaneously raise left arm and left leg to touch in midair. Hold. Lower arm and leg to stem. Repeat to other side.

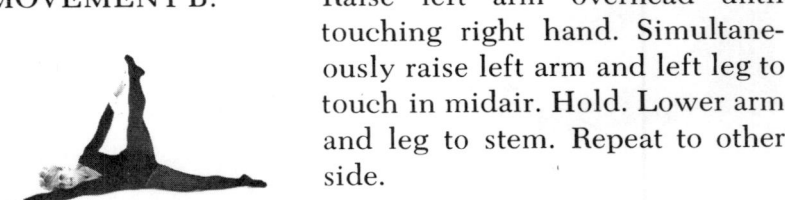

TO ATTAIN FITNESS
OR FOR WARM-UP: Ten on each side.

AS MAINTENANCE: Thirty on each side.

AREA: Abdomen—Spine

STEM POSITION 5:   Lie on back. Knees bent and together. Feet flat on floor. Arms out to sides, shoulder level.

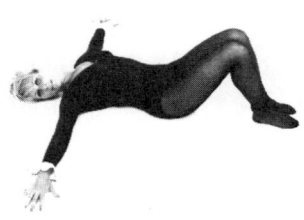

MOVEMENT A: Draw right knee to chest. Clasp knee with hands. Gently press knees closer to chest four times. On the fifth time, lift head up and try to touch knee to nose. Hold.

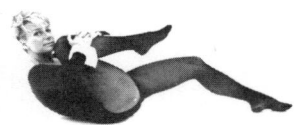

Lower head to floor, release knee to stem. Repeat sequence with left knee.

TO ATTAIN FITNESS
OR FOR WARM-UP: Repeat three times on each side.

AS MAINTENANCE: Gradually work up to six times on each side.

MOVEMENT B: Draw both knees to chest. Clasp knees with hands. Press knees closer to chest four times. The fifth time, lift head up and try to touch forehead to knees. Hold. Release head to floor, and knees to stem.

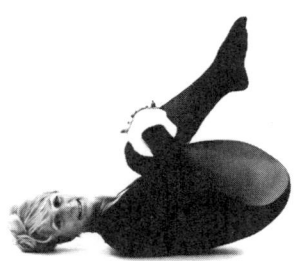

TO ATTAIN FITNESS
OR FOR WARM-UP: Repeat four times.

AS MAINTENANCE: Gradually work up to eight times.

MOVEMENT C: Slowly raise hips off floor. Hold hip-lift four counts. Slowly lower hips to floor. Support weight on your feet and shoulders. Try to increase the height of the hip-lifts.

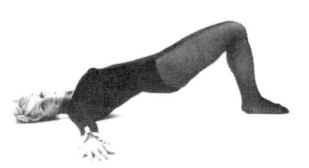

TO ATTAIN FITNESS
OR FOR WARM-UP: Repeat hip-lift six times.

68 DOCTOR SOLOMON

AS MAINTENANCE: Gradually work up to twelve times.

MOVEMENT D: 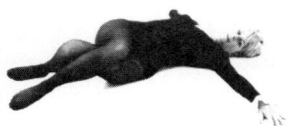 Cross right leg over left above the knee. Slowly press both knees toward the floor to the left side without lifting shoulders from floor. Bring legs back to center position. Repeat side press two times. Stop. Press knees to right side. Hold. Return knees to center. Repeat side press two times to right. Stop. Recross legs with left leg over right. Repeat sequence.

TO ATTAIN FITNESS
OR FOR WARM-UP: Repeat sequence four times.

AS MAINTENANCE: Gradually work up to twelve times.

AREA: Hips—Thighs—Buttocks

STEM POSITION 6: Stand with legs comfortably wide apart. Knees relaxed. Arms loosely down at sides.

The Master Plan   69

MOVEMENT A:

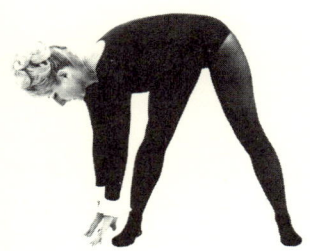

Bend down. Moving from right to left, try to touch hands to floor outside your right foot. Then bounce and touch your toes, bounce again and touch the floor between your feet. Bounce and move upper torso until you touch the outside of left foot. Stop. Slowly swing to upright position. Repeat bend and bounce, starting to the left side. Aim for four bounces before swinging up. Alternate sides.

TO ATTAIN FITNESS
OR FOR WARM-UP: Repeat sequence four times.

AS MAINTENANCE: Gradually work up to ten times.

MOVEMENT B:

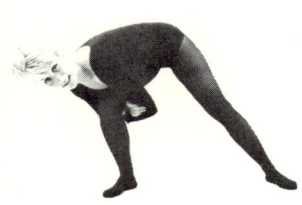

Bend right knee. Lunge over knee and grip arms together at elbows under knee. Hold. Keep both feet flat on floor, weight over right knee. Straighten up. Repeat deep lunge over left knee, gripping elbows under knees.

TO ATTAIN FITNESS
OR FOR WARM-UP: Alternate sides and repeat six times.

AS MAINTENANCE: Alternate sides and gradually work up to twelve times.

MOVEMENT C:

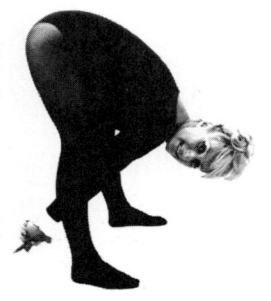

Bend forward. Clasp hands in front of you. Try to press hands to the floor between legs while swinging arms toward the back. In this position, bounce two times. Slowly straighten up and swing arms overhead. Bend knees and press hips forward. Bounce two times. Return to stem.

TO ATTAIN FITNESS
OR FOR WARM-UP: Repeat sequence four times.

AS MAINTENANCE: Gradually work up to twelve times.

MOVEMENT D:

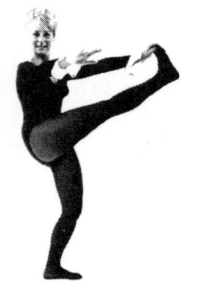

Extend arms front, waist high. Swing right leg up to left hand. Try to touch foot to hand in mid-air. Alternate legs and hands. Try to maintain a steady rhythm, with a pace comfortable for you.

TO ATTAIN FITNESS
OR FOR WARM-UP: Repeat eight times.

AS MAINTENANCE: Gradually work up to twenty times.

STEM POSITION 7: Stand erect. Feet together.

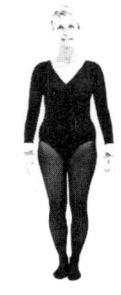

MOVEMENT A: √

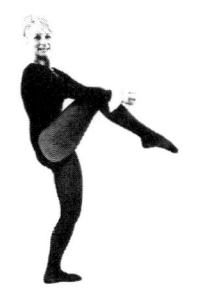

Clasp hands. Hold arms straight out front, approximately waist high. Bend right knee and raise knee between arms, toward chest. Lower leg to floor. Lift the left knee up between arms, toward chest.

TO ATTAIN FITNESS
OR FOR WARM-UP: Alternate legs and repeat ten times.

AS MAINTENANCE: Gradually work up to thirty times.

MOVEMENT B:

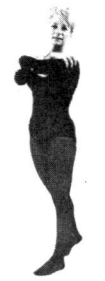

While walking briskly, vigorously swing arms back, shoulder level, on count one. Hold. On count two, bend elbows, swing arms forward until opposite hands clasp shoulders. Hold. Continue to alternate back arm swings with forward shoulder clasp.

TO ATTAIN FITNESS
OR FOR WARM-UP: Begin with twelve.

AS MAINTENANCE: Gradually work up to fifty.

MOVEMENT C: Keep feet together, knees relaxed, and arms loosely down at sides. Jump up and down. Try to land lightly on the balls of your feet, heels lightly touching floor. For variety, try the following in groups of ten: Jump forward and back; from side to side; in circles to right side, then left side.

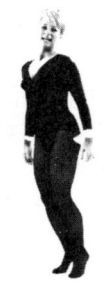

TO ATTAIN FITNESS
OR FOR WARM-UP: Twenty jumps.

AS MAINTENANCE: Gradually work up to two hundred.

Part III

6 Area of Concentration: The Abdomen

The Problem. Have you ever noticed that a good portion of the population, male as well as female, appears slightly pregnant? It is the unusual silhouette that reveals a taut, tight tummy, held firmly in place. Watch your favorite celebrities on television or in the movies. They've learned to angle their bodies so that abdomens are always front on—even when the upper torso is side to the camera. This figure fault afflicts all ages, teenagers through adults of both sexes. Being slender is no insurance; in fact, it makes the protuberance just that much more noticeable.

Why should this be the great American profile? Mostly because we are all neglecting appropriate exercise and appropriate diet. As we become more and more a nation of button pushers, our posture declines. Primitive men and women who carried their burdens on their heads stood tall so that every muscle bore a portion of that burden. No drooping abdomens there. And they didn't wear girdles, either. Artificial assistance makes unused muscles even lazier. Would you work if you could rely on someone else to support you?

The Program. To develop a strong, natural abdominal girdle of your own muscles, you must increase the circulation in this area and burn up the excess stored fat. Taut stomach muscles can be evolved by correcting poor posture and by remedial exercising. During the day, as you sit, stand, or work, you can exercise these muscles by constantly pulling them in tightly against your spine. Remind yourself to do this so often that it becomes a habit. The more you tighten your abdominal muscles, the tighter and stronger they become.

The program for concentration on the abdominals includes activity to work on the problems of circulation and stored fat. It is also planned so that all the muscles—upper, lower, and oblique—in the abdomen are included. You will note that you do some of the exercises in several ways. This places stress on the specific muscles in turn.

Technique Tips. By sitting up with your knees bent (hip flex position), you protect your back and help yourself to balance. You want to work your abdominal muscles, not your back muscles in these exercises.

At first you may find a little bit of trouble in sitting up from the stem position. In that case, begin the exercise from the upright seated position with knees bent, but roll down as directed. Sit up any way you can. Your abdominal muscles will soon strengthen so that you can follow the directions to the letter. As the muscles strengthen, increase your demands on them in the sit-ups by striving for a slow, steady, prolonged pull.

Curling your body is tremendously important. You leave the floor with your head first, next your shoulders, and finally your back. You curl down in reverse order, with your back first, then your shoulders, then your head. Curling should be a slow and fluid movement, not a rapid series of jerks.

The Abdomen

EXERCISES

STEM POSITION 1:

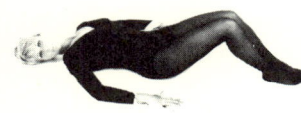

Lie down on your back on floor, knees bent and together, feet flat on floor.

MOVEMENT A:

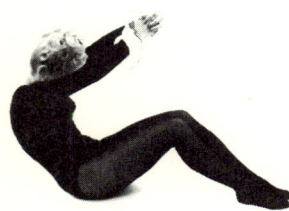

Clasp hands over head, elbows slightly bent. Slowly curl head, shoulders, and back from floor to upright sitting position. When sitting up, let each knee open out to the side—soles and heels pressed together. Bend forward, bouncing down two times toward the toes, until hands are over them. Bring knees together. Slowly roll down to floor, chin on chest, hands forward, until shoulders touch floor. Then return hands over head. Begin with five times; increase gradually to twelve.

MOVEMENT B:

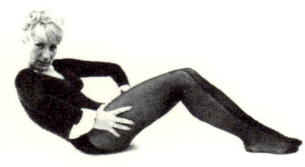

Place hands on thighs. Keep knees pressed together. Curl head, shoulders, and back from floor to full sit-up. Hold. Slowly uncurl to the floor. Hold. Begin with five times; increase gradually to ten.

MOVEMENT C:

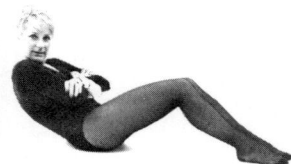

Grasp arms at elbows close to body. Keep knees pressed together. Curl to sitting position. Hold. Slowly uncurl to the floor. Hold. Begin with four; increase gradually to twelve.

MOVEMENT D:

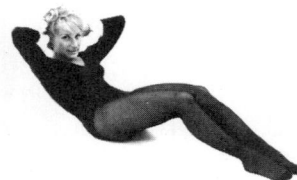

Lace fingers behind neck, elbows flat to floor. Roll up to sitting position. Hold. Slowly roll back down to floor. Hold. Begin with five; increase gradually to fifteen.

STEM POSITION 2:

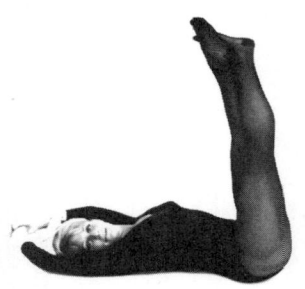

Lie on floor. Raise legs toward ceiling, knees straight, toes pointed, ankles crossed. Hands clasped over head on floor.

The Abdomen 79

MOVEMENT A:

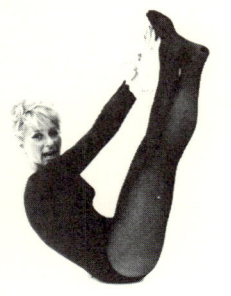

Curl head, chest, and shoulders up from floor; try to touch hands to ankles or toes. Hold. Slowly uncurl to floor. Begin with four; increase gradually to twelve.

MOVEMENT B:

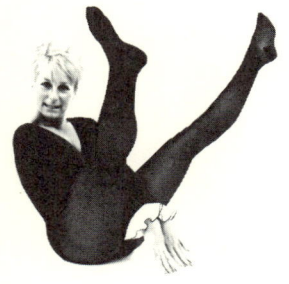

Simultaneously roll head, chest, and shoulders off floor as legs separate in a wide V. Come to upright position and stabilize on buttocks with hands touching floor between legs. Hold momentarily. Roll down to floor and bring legs together to stem position. Begin with four; increase gradually to twelve.

STEM POSITION 3:

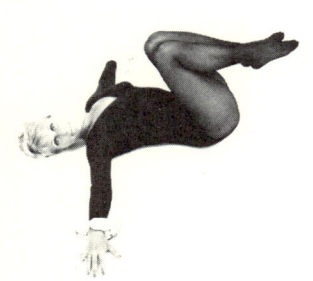

Lie on floor, knees bent to chest. Arms out shoulder level, palms to floor.

80 DOCTOR SOLOMON

MOVEMENT A:

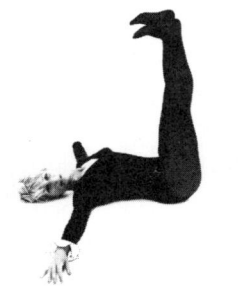

Slowly extend both legs to ceiling, toes pointed. Pause. With legs up, flex heels and point toes two times. Hold. Slowly lower knees to chest. If knees bend at first, don't force full extension. Begin with six; increase gradually to sixteen.

MOVEMENT B:

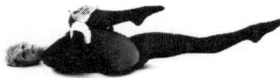

Lace fingers; place hands on right knee and press to chest. Slowly extend left leg low over floor. Flex and point foot. Simultaneously bend left knee to chest as right leg extends low over floor. Change hands to left knee. Flex and point right foot. Continue to alternate. Begin with eight horizontal bicycle stretches; increase gradually to twenty.

MOVEMENT C:

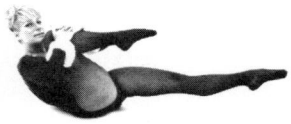

Repeat bicycle stretch. While one knee is pressed to chest, slowly curl chest off floor. Try to touch chin to knee. Lower chest and head to floor. Change legs. Repeat chin-to-knee press on the other side. Begin with four; increase gradually to twelve.

The Abdomen 81

MOVEMENT D:

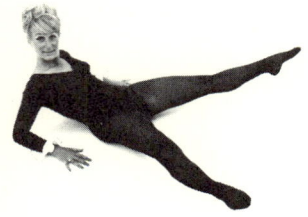

Place arms beside body. Keep knees to chest. Curl head, chest, and back off floor. With weight on forearms, slowly extend both legs low over floor, toes pointed. Hold. Separate legs to sides in wide spread. Hold. Bring legs together front. Hold. Return legs to chest. Repeat sequence four times; work up gradually to twelve.

STEM POSITION 4: Lie on floor, knees bent, hip-width apart, feet flat on floor.

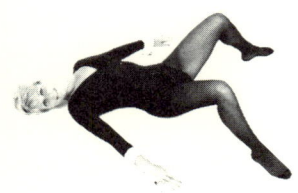

MOVEMENT A:

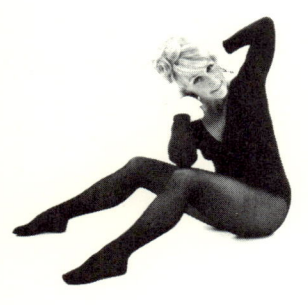

Lace fingers behind head, elbows flat to floor. Slowly roll head, shoulders, and back off floor until upright. Twist chest and touch right elbow to outside of left knee. Slowly roll down to floor. Repeat roll-up and twist and touch left elbow to outside of right knee. Slowly roll down to floor. Begin with four; increase gradually to twelve.

MOVEMENT B:

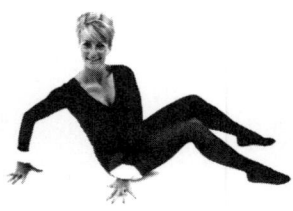

Clasp hands overhead on floor. Swing up to sitting position and twist chest to right side. Try to place palms on floor by hips. Hold. Clasp hands, roll back down to floor. Repeat sit-up and twist to left side. Hold. Slowly roll down to floor. Begin with six; increase gradually to twelve.

STEM POSITION 5:

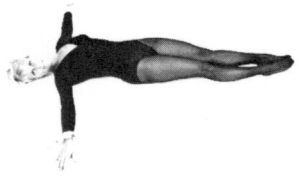

Lie on floor, legs straight and together, arms out shoulder level, palms to floor.

MOVEMENT:

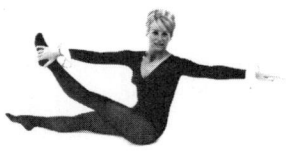

Simultaneously swing upper torso off floor as left leg lifts. Twist chest left and touch right hand to left foot in midair. Hold. Slowly release body to stem position. Repeat sit-up, with left hand to right foot in midair. Hold. Begin with six sit-ups; increase gradually to twelve.

7 Area of Concentration: The Arms and Chest

The Problem. Unless a woman is involved in sports or heavy physical work, her upper arms will tend to become flabby and weak. It is my observation that Americans tend to use their arms less not just as they become adults, but also as a form of physical expression when walking, talking, or social dancing.

The resulting flabbiness is actually due to muscle atrophy. When you exercise just one group of muscles over and over, you neglect others in the same area. The neglected ones atrophy from inactivity. In the case of arm muscles, this is particularly noticeable among women. Men have always had the convenience of shirt sleeves and jackets as camouflage.

Along with sagging upper arms go sagging busts. The same exercise that strengthens the arms will strengthen the pectoral muscles that underlie the bustline. Breasts are glands, not muscles; and despite those cleavage ads in the backs of the magazines, you cannot stimulate their development. What you can do to make them *appear* larger is to strengthen the muscles underneath the glands. While men are not concerned with their bustlines, the exercises work for them as well by correcting poor shoulder posture. The final motivation for exercising the arms is to relieve the shoulder tension that plagues so many people.

The Program. To exercise every muscle in the arms, you must learn to reach, to flex, to press, and to make circling motions. This brings into play muscles in the under and back parts of the arm that are generally inactive. You will feel the effects down across your chest as the pectoral muscles work.

Technique Tips. Some of these exercises have the letter W beside them. That is a signal to you that you may increase the demands on your muscles by doing these exercises with an equal weight in each hand. I advise using a one-pound weight, available at most sporting-goods stores, but two one-pound cans of anything in your kitchen will serve as well. If your cupboard is bare, two books will do.

It is important to put all of the action into the arms and shoulders as directed. Do not move any other part of the body unless the exercise direction explicitly tells you to do so.

EXERCISES

STEM POSITION 1: Sit on floor. Arms extended at sides, shoulders level, palms down. Assume one of the three basic positions:

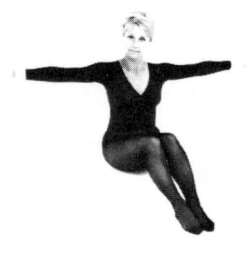

Tailor-fashion—legs crossed, with feet under knees; Diamond pattern—knees out to sides, soles and heels pressed together; Hip-flexed position—knees together and bent, feet flat on floor.

The Arms and Chest

MOVEMENT A:

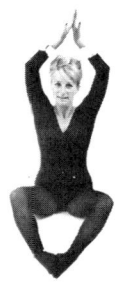

Slowly raise arms over head until knuckles touch. Hold. Turn hands until palms touch. Hold. Turn hands until knuckles touch. Hold. Slowly lower arms to shoulder level. The pattern is to touch knuckles, palms, knuckles. Lower to stem position. Keep elbows straight. Begin with ten raises; gradually increase to thirty.

MOVEMENT B:

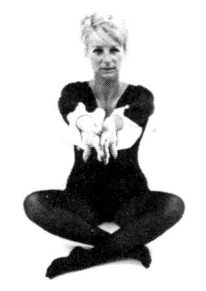

Swing arms to front, elbows straight, until knuckles touch. Hold. Turn hands till palms touch. Hold. Turn hands until knuckles touch. Hold. Swing arms out to sides shoulder level, palms open and facing back. Repeat the forward swing, with the "knuckles, palms, knuckles" pattern. Begin with ten; gradually increase to thirty.

MOVEMENT C:

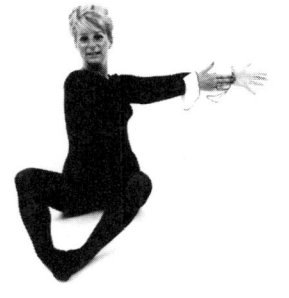

Rotate arms until palms face front. Swing right arm across chest until palms touch. Hold. Swing right arm back to side. Swing left arm across chest until palms touch. Hold. Swing left arm to original position. Keep both arms straight throughout. Nonmoving arm remains stationary at shoulder level. Keep upper torso stationary and facing front. Alternate arm swings. Begin with ten; gradually increase to thirty.

STEM POSITION 2: Sit on floor. Assume one position—tailor, diamond, or hip-flexed. Fingers resting on shoulders, elbows out to sides, shoulder level.

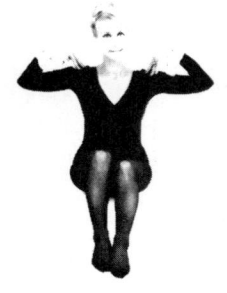

MOVEMENT A: Press elbows together until touching. Hold. Release elbows back to open position. Hold. Try to keep elbows shoulder level throughout exercise. Begin with ten; increase gradually to thirty.

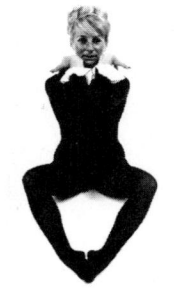

MOVEMENT B: Lift elbows up behind head until knuckles touch. Hold. Press elbows down to sides toward waist. Hold. Begin with eight; increase gradually to sixteen.

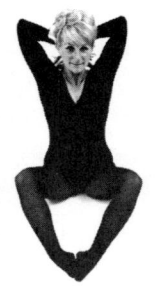

The Arms and Chest   87

MOVEMENT C:

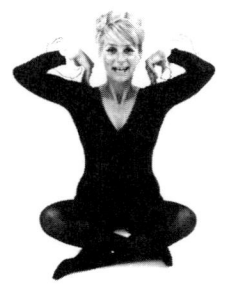

Rotate both elbows in a circle. Begin by lowering elbows down to sides, touching waist. Point elbows foward and up. Press elbows back to shoulder level. Lower elbows to waist. Lead with both elbows. Continue to make big circles in the air. Begin with four circles forward, then four backward. Increase total circles gradually to ten in each direction.

STEM POSITION 3:

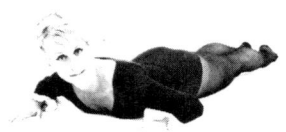

Lie face down on floor. Legs together, toes pointed. Arms directly under shoulders, elbows bent. Palms flat on floor.

MOVEMENT A:

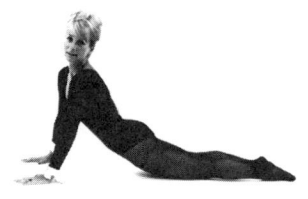

Slowly raise only the front part of your body off floor. Lift the head, chest, stomach, and hips up until arms are straight. Hold. Keep back straight. Slowly return to stem position. Repeat four times; increase gradually to twelve.

MOVEMENT B:

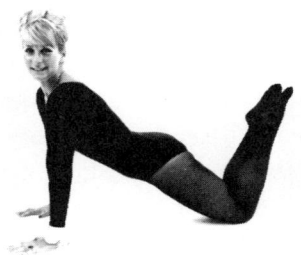

Bend knees with heels toward buttocks. Slowly push torso off floor until resting on knees. When arms are straight, hold position for three seconds. Slowly lower body to stem position. Hold body rigid during lifting and lowering. Begin with four; increase gradually to twelve.

STEM POSITION 4:

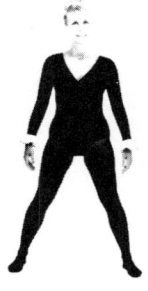

Stand erect, legs wide apart. Feet flat on floor. Arms at sides.

MOVEMENT A:

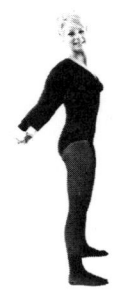

Clasp hands behind back at buttocks. Slowly pull arms back and away from body. Hold. Return clasped hands to buttocks. Repeat eight times; increase gradually to twenty.

The Arms and Chest   89

MOVEMENT B: Clasp hands. Arms down in front of body. Slowly lift arms overhead. Hold. Bend elbows, lower hands behind head to neck. Hold. Lift arms straight over head. Hold. Lower arms straight down. Repeat ten times; increase gradually to thirty.

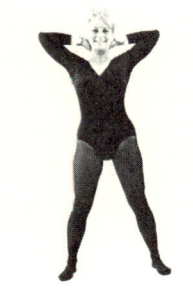

MOVEMENT C: Bend forward from hips. Bring arms to front, shoulder level. Alternating arms, swim stroke forward, arm-over-arm. Keep reaching forward as far as possible. After ten strokes front, turn upper body to right and complete ten strokes to right side. Turn torso over to left side for ten more strokes. Return front and repeat series. Complete thirty strokes. Work up gradually to sixty strokes.

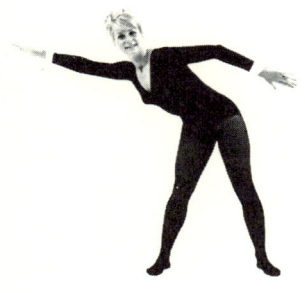

MOVEMENT D: Bend knees slightly forward. Alternating arms, swim the backstroke. Keep arms straight and close to head as they stroke back. Begin with twelve backstrokes; increase gradually to sixty.

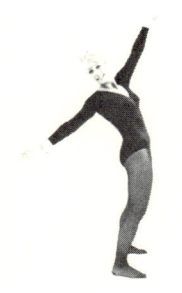

8 Area of Concentration: The Back

The Problem. Have you seen what's going on behind your back? Unless you regularly stand before a three-way mirror, you may have no idea that fleshy fat deposits are disfiguring the region from your shoulders to your waist. For some reason, what you can't see doesn't worry you. I have found that people complain about their backs only when they ache. It is the one area of the body where vanity does not seem to be involved—only comfort.

The discomfort in your back arises when your back has become weak and inflexible because the muscles in your spine have not been fully stretched. Or you may have a physical ailment that has contributed directly to your back problem. Whatever the cause, the full range of movement has been reduced.

The Program. You know your own back best. Do you suffer from special physical or medical problems with your spine? If so, proceed to Chapter 15 after you get your doctor's approval. Those continuing with this chapter should also consult with their doctors about these exercises before beginning.

The exercises themselves are separated into two sections: one for those who want to increase their back flexibility and strength; the other for those who wish to slim down or firm up a fleshy back. I advise doing both so that you are lithe, limber, and attractive coming and going.

Technique Tips. Easy does it. Ease your torso up from a forward bending position to an upright one. Never snap it up quickly. Think of your spine uncurling slowly, one vertebra at a time. Straighten your back gradually, starting with the lower back, the mid-back, and finally the shoulders. The head lifts up last.

You should not be tense doing this; but if after the initial warm-up exercise your back does remain tense, bend both knees slightly for any of the exercises that follow that involve the side, forward bouncing, or bending and bobbing. This adjustment will place less demand on your back until it has loosened up.

INCREASED FLEXIBILITY AND STRENGTH FOR THE BACK

STEM POSITION 1: Sit on floor with soles and heels pressed against each other, knees out to sides. Lean forward and grasp ankles; elbows rest outside of knees.

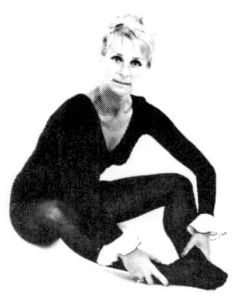

MOVEMENT A:

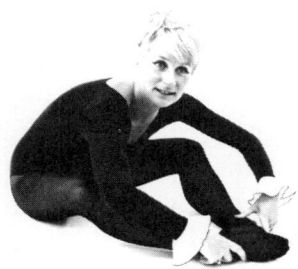

Drop head, round the back. Slowly bounce forward, head as close to heels as you can get. Remain in forward position. Continue to bounce over feet four times. Slowly release upright to stem position. Repeat low back stretch four times; work up gradually to ten.

MOVEMENT B:

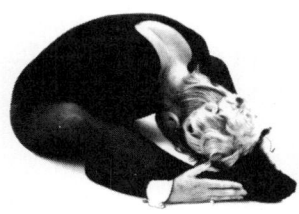

Pass arms under inside of thighs, hands under legs gripping ankles from outside on each side. Bend trunk forward and down. Bounce forward gently four times. Let head drop forward in an effort to touch heels. Return to stem position. As you limber up, your elbows should touch the floor. Begin with a few seconds of stretching daily; increase gradually to one minute.

STEM POSITION 2:

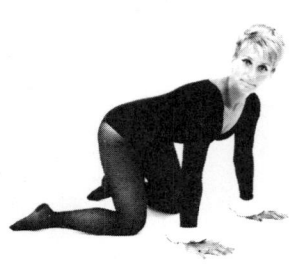

Kneel on hands and knees. Insteps are pressed to floor. Elbows straight, palms flat on floor. Weight forward over hands.

MOVEMENT A:

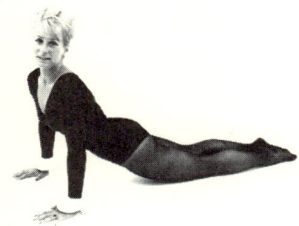

Slowly push backward away from arms until buttocks rest on heels. Head down. Hold. Slowly stretch torso forward between arms until knees are straight. Head back. Hold. Return to stem. Repeat four times; work up gradually to twelve.

MOVEMENT B:

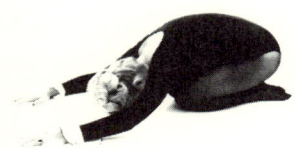

Slowly push trunk back until buttocks rest on heels. Hold. Bring both arms back to rest loosely on floor at sides. Lower forehead until touching floor. Hold this position. Breathe slowly until you feel relaxed. Stop if you feel dizzy.

STEM POSITION 3:

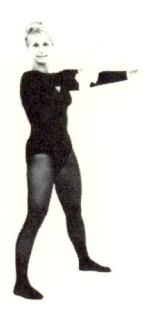

Stand, legs wide apart, knees slightly bent. Hands clasped behind back.

MOVEMENT A:

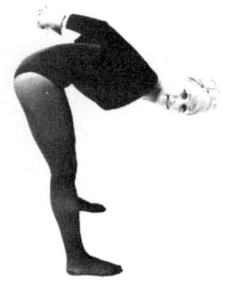

Bend forward from hips. Keep head up and bounce upper body down toward floor in six bounces. Then drop arms loosely toward floor. Let head and whole upper body hang. Bounce six times gently in this relaxed position. Slowly return to stem. Repeat head-up bounce, alternating with head-down bounce three times; increase gradually to six times.

MOVEMENT B:

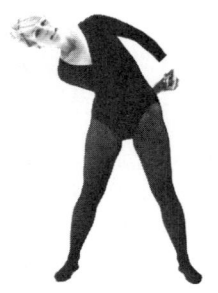

Simultaneously bend trunk over to right side as you pull clasped hands as far as possible to left side. Bounce four times, stretching down on right side. Return to center. Repeat to other side. Alternate sides. Begin with four sets; work up gradually to eight.

FIRMER CONTOUR FOR THE BACK

STEM POSITION 1:

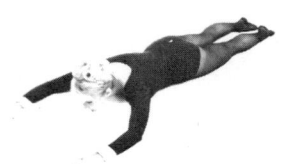

Lie on stomach. Legs together and straight. Insteps pressed to floor. Arms extended front, palms down, chin on floor.

The Back

MOVEMENT A:

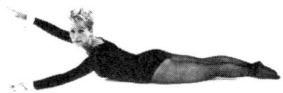

Slowly raise right arm forward and up. Hold. Lower arm to floor. Slowly raise left arm front and up. Hold. Return to stem. Do not roll chest from side to side as arm raises. Alternate sides. Begin with eight; work up gradually to twenty.

MOVEMENT B:

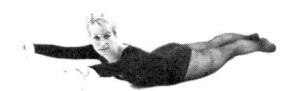

Slowly raise both arms and head off floor. Hold. Slowly lower to stem. Begin with six; increase gradually to twelve.

MOVEMENT C:

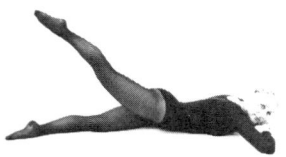

Slowly raise right leg off floor, knee straight. Hold. Lower. Raise left leg off floor. Hold. Slowly lower to stem. Begin with eight; increase to sixteen.

MOVEMENT D:

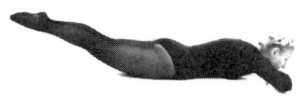

Slowly raise both legs up. Hold. Release. Begin with six; increase gradually to twelve.

MOVEMENT E:

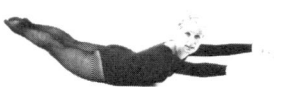

Tighten buttock muscles. Slowly raise arms and legs at the same time off floor. Keep head between raised arms. Release to stem. Begin with four; increase gradually to twelve.

STEM POSITION 2: Kneel with knees apart. Hands flat on floor in line with shoulders.

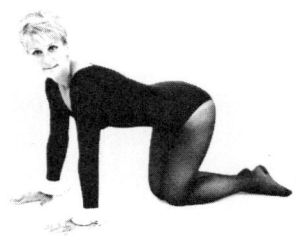

MOVEMENT A:

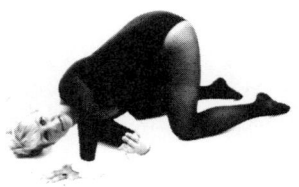

Stretch right arm out shoulder level to right side. Keep arm straight. Turn head to follow movement. Hold. Bend elbow. Twist arm downward into space between left hand and knee. Try to touch floor with right ear and shoulder. Release upright with arm out to side. Repeat complete movement four times on one side. Repeat on other side. Begin with five to each side; work up gradually to ten.

MOVEMENT B:

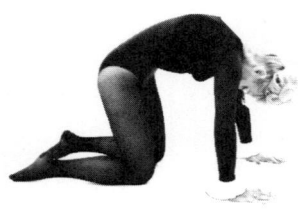

Slowly pull stomach in, and round your back high to a hump position. Head drops down. Hold. Release to stem. Repeat five times; work up gradually to twelve. Keep arms straight throughout.

The Back   97

MOVEMENT C:

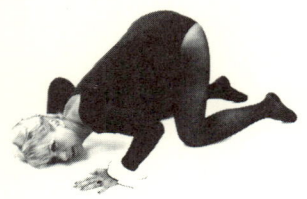

Slowly bend elbows out and lower chest to floor. Try to touch right cheek to floor between arms. Hold. Release to stem. Alternate sides. Begin with six; work up gradually to twelve.

STEM POSITION 3:

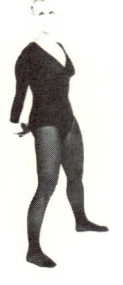

Stand erect. Legs wide apart. Stretch arms forward, shoulder level, palms turned up.

MOVEMENT A:

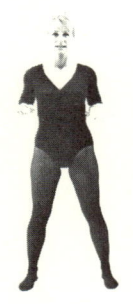

Bend elbows and pull arms straight back until hands are on each side of chest. Hold. Stretch arms forward, arms straight. Hold. Keep arms close to body on backward pull. Repeat eight times; increase gradually to twenty.

98   DOCTOR SOLOMON

MOVEMENT B: Bend elbows, place fingertips on shoulders to the front. Hold. Lift both elbows forward and up toward ceiling. Hold. Lower elbows to body. Hold. Stretch arms forward to stem. Repeat eight times; work up gradually to sixteen.

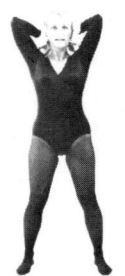

9 Area of Concentration: The Buttocks

The Problem. Ogden Nash said it best in his poem about women wearing slacks: "Have you seen yourself retreating?" Well, have you? Do you suffer from baggy buttocks?

I am not including the hips and thighs in this section. They come later on.

Excessive weight and lack of exercise, together with the "sititis" common to modern living, aggravate the droop in the derriere. Sitting deactivates the buttock muscles by keeping them inactive and constricting the circulation in the area. As I have repeated many times in this book, to keep muscles healthy, good circulation is necessary. Where weight is a problem, fat buttocks are a large part of the problem.

The Program. Within the program for the buttocks, you will find, first of all, exercises to uplift your derriere by strengthening and firming the large buttock muscles. Then you will have some other exercises which also firm and strengthen them, but also serve to increase the circulation

100   DOCTOR SOLOMON

in the area, thus helping to break up the fatty tissue. Then there are multipurpose exercises that involve both the buttocks and the hips.

Technique Tips. As you do these exercises, whenever one leg is crossing over the torso, your head should be turning in the opposite direction. This will help you to keep your shoulders pinned to the floor, increasing the effect of the exercise.

Deep massage can hasten the results of these buttock exercises. Before you start, give your buttocks a mini massage by cupping your hands under each cheek and pinching or kneading fifteen times with your knuckles. Or you may massage your flesh with fingers and thumb.

Another way of increasing the effect of these exercises is to do the ones marked P in a swimming pool. Just be sure that you hold onto the pool ladder, a corner, or the coping for support. The resistance of the water will force you to push harder, your muscles will become stronger, and you will feel more relaxed when you have completed your exercises.

EXERCISES

STEM POSITION 1: Lie on stomach. Legs straight and together, insteps pressed to floor. Hands on floor either under chin or under hips.

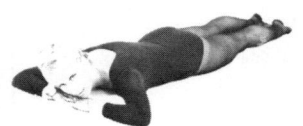

MOVEMENT A:

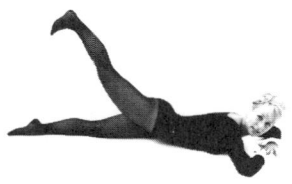

Lift right leg high off floor, toes pointed. Hold. Lower leg to stem. Lift left leg high off floor. Hold. Lower to stem. Repeat lift and add a flex and point to each foot when in midair. Alternate legs ten times; work up gradually to twenty.

MOVEMENT B:

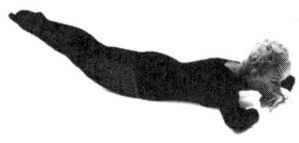

Lift both legs high off floor. Hold. Lower to stem. Keep knees straight and toes pointed. Tighten buttocks as legs lift, release buttocks as legs lower. Begin with five; increase gradually to twelve.

MOVEMENT C:

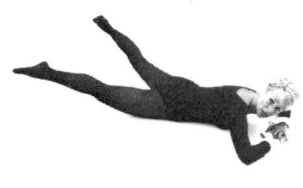

Lift both legs slightly off floor. Hold. Separate legs and scissor them wide to the side. Hold. Bring legs together. Hold. Open legs on count of one and close on two. Keep counting in this fashion until legs are together on eight. Lower legs to stem. Repeat sequence three times; increase gradually to six.

STEM POSITION 2:

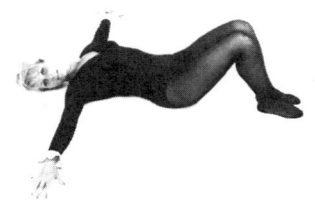

Lie on back. Knees bent and together. Feet flat on floor. Arms outstretched, shoulder level, palms to floor.

MOVEMENT A:

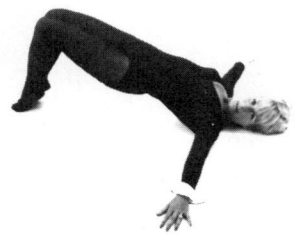

Tense buttock muscles. Lift buttocks high off floor. Hold. While in high lift position, raise heels off floor, then lower heels to floor, eight times. Lower buttocks to stem. Repeat sequence four times; increase gradually to ten.

MOVEMENT B:

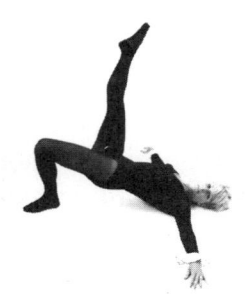

Lift buttocks off floor. Hold. Raise right leg toward ceiling. Hold. Bend knee. Lower buttocks to floor. Return to stem. Repeat sequence to other side. Alternate sides. Begin with four; increase gradually to twelve.

MOVEMENT C:

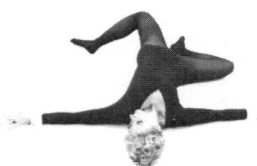

Separate legs, keep knees bent. Lift buttocks high off floor. Hold. Twist trunk to left side and lower left hip to floor. Try to press both knees to left side on floor. Hold. Return to stem. Lift buttocks high off floor. Hold. Twist trunk to right side and lower right hip to floor. Try to press knees to right side on floor. Hold. Return to stem. Alternate sides. Repeat six times; increase gradually to fourteen.

The Buttocks   103

STEM POSITION 3: Sit on floor, legs straight and together. Lean back; rest on hands.

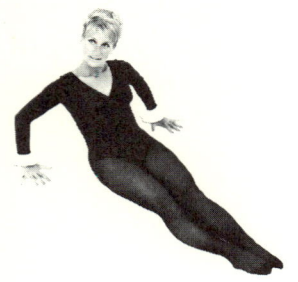

MOVEMENT A: Lift right leg off floor. Cross right leg over left until foot touches floor. Hold. Lift right leg up and return to stem. Repeat with left leg to right side. Keep legs straight and chest front as hips twist to each side. Alternate sides. Begin with eight; increase gradually to sixteen.

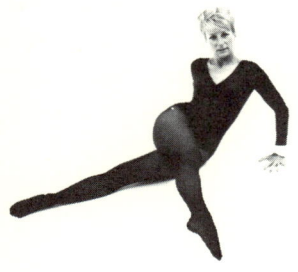

MOVEMENT B: Lift right leg off floor. Cross right leg high over left until right foot touches floor. Hold. Swing right leg up again and far out to right side until foot touches floor. Hold. Slide leg back on floor to stem. Cross left leg over right until left foot touches floor. Hold. Swing left leg up again and far out to left side until foot touches floor. Hold. Slide leg back on floor to stem. Alternate sides. Begin with four; increase gradually to twelve.

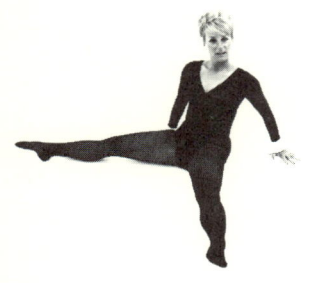

MOVEMENT C:

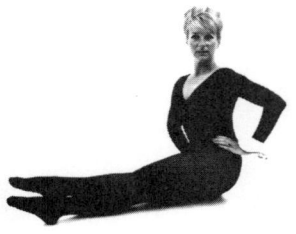

Place hands on hips. "Walk" across room on buttocks. Roll from hip to hip as you lift opposite leg and push it forward. Keep legs straight. Move with waist pulled up off hips. Try moving forward for one minute. Repeat, moving backward, one minute.

STEM POSITION 4:

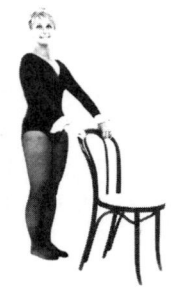

Stand erect, feet together. Hold back of chair with both hands for support. Do not lean against chair. Keep upper torso facing front.

MOVEMENT A:
P

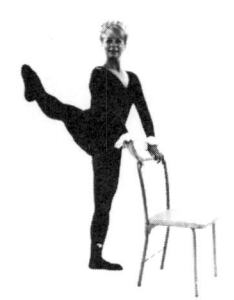

Swing right leg out to right side. Lower legs and swing to left side. Toes lightly brush floor between each swing. Try to swing leg as high as you can to each side. Supporting leg remains straight. Begin with ten to each side; increase gradually to thirty.

The Buttocks

MOVEMENT B:
P

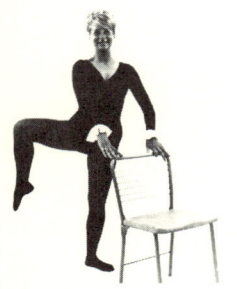

Lift right knee to waist. Hold. With knee waist high and bent, slowly open knee out to right side. Hold. Return knee to front. Hold. Repeat side-front action four times before lowering to stem. Anchor leg remains straight. Repeat to other side. Increase gradually to twelve to each side.

MOVEMENT C:
P

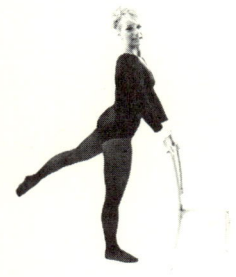

Swing right leg directly back and as high as possible, keeping leg straight. Keep toes pointed and lift leg high for two counts. Lower leg to stem. Repeat to other side. Alternate sides. Begin with eight; increase gradually to twenty.

10 Area of Concentration: The Feet and Ankles

The Problem. You are always stepping on your feet. All the weight you have is concentrated on one foot or the other every time you move. That's quite a burden to bear when you stop to think about it. No wonder feet revolt by feeling heavy or by aching and swelling.

There is help for your feet within their muscles. What connects foot bones is muscle tissue, and that can be strengthened so that your feet are better equipped to hold you up during your day's activities. Weak foot muscles and weak feet contribute to overall fatigue. When your feet hurt, you hurt—all over. Learning how to avoid this hurt will contribute to an overall sense of well-being.

The Program. You will be surprised at how much there is to exercise in the limited vicinity of your foot. The program will help you maintain or develop flexibility in the ankles, toes, and the backs of your heels—an area you probably never consider exists. You will discover how to stretch your foot muscles properly so that weakness and inflexibility are eliminated. Doing these foot exercises regularly can alleviate many of your foot problems.

The Feet and Ankles

Technique Tips for Foot Care. Your feet spend much of the time encased in a close-fitting leather prison. In addition, women's feet are often wrapped in nylon, a nonbreathing, nonabsorptive material. It would be thoughtful of you to release your feet from their prisons of leather and nylon and let them go bare. Letting air touch your feet as frequently as possible does them a world of good. So does walking barefoot on sand or grass.

Before you go to bed, grasp your big toes and rotate them slowly in both directions. This keeps them flexible.

Let one foot rub the other. Rubbing the tops and soles of one foot with your other foot is soothing. Or if you prefer, massage by hand.

A real treat for feet is a soak in a quart of lukewarm water with a bath oil or Epsom salt added.

Here are some suggestions for relieving swollen feet:

Keep an extra pair of comfortable, properly fitting shoes on hand so that you may change during the day.

Prop your feet higher than your hips from time to time. This is an antigravity position that eases the flow of blood and helps prevent swelling of the legs.

Try a rejuvenating lower-leg massage. Begin at your ankles and use both hands in a firm patting-slapping action. Rub all the way up to your knees.

Slip off your shoes. Wiggle your toes briskly, then spread them apart, separating them as far as you can.

Always buy your shoes late in the day when your feet are most swollen. Then the shoes will fit at the time of the day when your feet are most swollen. When trying on shoes, simulate the motions of your daily activities as much as possible.

The following exercises for feet and ankles should be done barefoot.

108   DOCTOR SOLOMON

EXERCISES

STEM POSITION 1:   Stand, feet parallel, slightly apart, and flat on the floor.

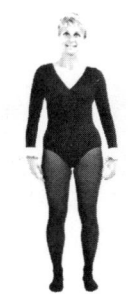

MOVEMENT A: With weight on right foot, vigorously shake left foot at ankle. See how limp and free your foot can feel. Repeat with right foot, ten times on each side.

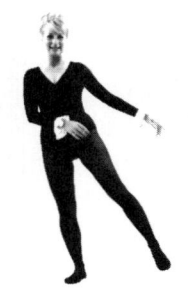

MOVEMENT B: Put weight on right foot. Slowly lift left heel off floor until resting on toes. Hold. Slowly lower heel to floor. Repeat heel lift to other side. Begin with eight; increase gradually to sixteen.

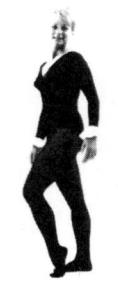

The Feet and Ankles 109

MOVEMENT C:

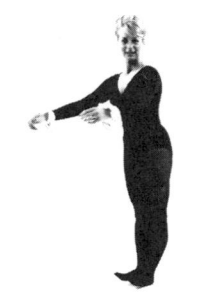

Slowly, with weight on both feet, rise up to toes. Hold. Lower to floor. Hold. Rock back on heels. Hold. Lower to floor. Alternate toe rises with heel rocking. Begin with six; increase gradually to twelve.

MOVEMENT D:

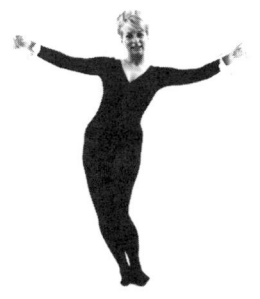

Bend both knees. Roll both feet over to right side. Hold. Roll both feet over to left side. Hold. Keep knees bent during rolls. Upper body remains still. Roll from edge to edge continuously six times; increase gradually to twelve.

STEM POSITION 2:

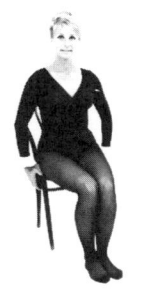

Sit on edge of chair, legs together and relaxed, feet flat on floor. Hold chair sides when necessary.

MOVEMENT A:

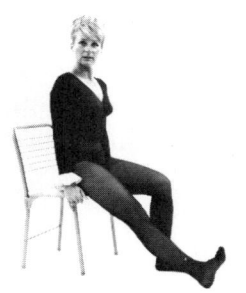

Extend right foot forward. Rest heel on floor, toes pointing up. Hold. Point toes sharply down to floor with strong flex. Hold two counts. Continue this heel-and-toe motion six times. Return foot to stem position. Repeat to other side. Increase gradually to twelve on each side.

MOVEMENT B:

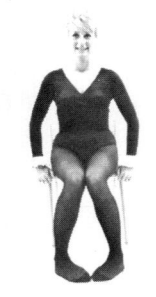

Push heels out hard in opposite directions. Toes will touch. Then swivel toes out, away from each other. Continue to "heel-and-toe" until legs are wide apart. Return to stem position by reversing movement. Bring heels, then toes, together. Begin with six; increase gradually to twelve.

STEM POSITION 3:

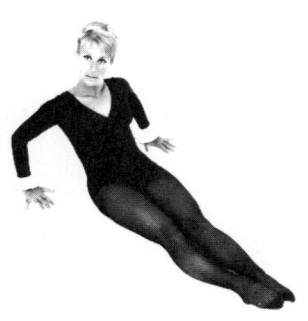

Sit on floor, bend right leg. Hands behind body on floor for support.

The Feet and Ankles

MOVEMENT A:

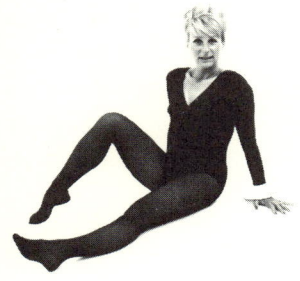

Slap sole of right foot against floor ten times. Slap right heel against floor ten times. Slap sole, then heel, six times. Repeat with left foot. Alternating sides, slap entire foot flat to floor ten times.

MOVEMENT B:

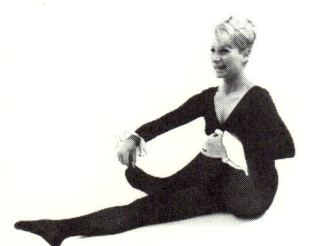

Rest left leg on right thigh. With right hand, loosen up each toe by making small circles with each one. Reverse direction. Repeat with right leg on left thigh.

MOVEMENT C:

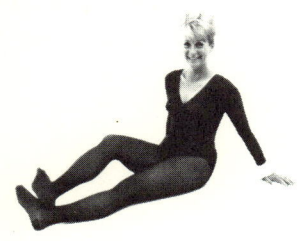

Foot-on-foot massage. Extend left leg. Use your right heel to knead and rub all over left foot. Move heel gently over instep, to base of toes, down along side area by each anklebone. Cover entire foot area. Repeat to other side.

11 Area of Concentration: The Hips

The Problem. In the case of hips, your problem may be in the genes. Do pictures of your family show a group of people with heavy hips? You may have inherited the tendency. I am here to tell you that the tendency can be thwarted. You need not accumulate fat (or cellulite, if you prefer) around your hips. Technically speaking, your hips are that area of your body between the waist and the buttocks.

The hip area is reducible with a proper combination of exercise and diet (see **Dr. Solomon's Easy, No-Risk Diet**). I would say that 10 percent of all the obese women I have treated have had heavy hips. Those who took my prescriptions for their eating problems and their activity problem lost weight and inches in eight out of ten cases by maintaining the dual regimen of hip exercise and diet *for one month.*

The usual reasons for flabbiness and spread in the hip region are: weakened muscles resulting from inactivity, artificial support, improper diet, and sedentary living. These can be complicated by recent childbirth.

The best time to seek hip control is when you first notice you are beginning to spread. If you manage to avoid the heavy pads that can build up, your job will be eased, and so will maintenance of your proper silhouette.

The Program. The program for hips is designed to activate the large muscles in hip and buttock area. This changes the contour of the hips, but you will derive a double benefit. You are involving your buttocks and thighs in inch-reducing as well. The exercises accelerate muscle activity, increase circulation, and strengthen your muscles, as all good exercises should.

Before you begin, it is important to overcome hip-joint stiffness. You can do this by isolating your hips and forcing them to move freely. Hip activity through exercise is a toning process, and you can help overcome the stiffness by a deep kneading massage.

My patients report to me that they have the best control when they do hip exercises from a floor position. They find this leaves them free to concentrate on their in-depth exercising without fear of losing their balance. I gladly pass this practical observation along to you.

Technique Tips. Take time out during these exercises to check your body position. In hip exercise especially, you must eliminate as much extraneous movement as possible. Shifting your weight or changing your body position may cause muscle cramping and/or improper exercising. It's worth taking the time to check so that you obtain the results you desire.

Your mind can consciously control your freedom of motion. Try using it as you exercise by thinking "Hips . . . loosen up . . . become freer . . . activate . . . become more a part of me." You will discover a new sense of your hips belonging to your body and of an ability to do something about them.

Do you remember in working the exercises for your

buttocks that your turned your head to the opposite direction of your working leg? Doing the same thing with the hip exercises also aids your balance, increases resistance, and adds to your comfort. So remember to turn your head in opposition to the movement of your leg.

EXERCISES

STEM POSITION 1:

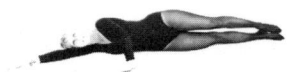

Lie on right side. Head resting on shoulder and outstretched arm. Left hand front, palm on floor for support, legs straight.

MOVEMENT A:

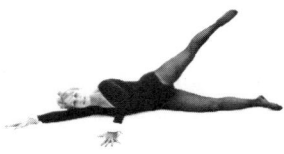

Lift left leg and make a complete circle in the air. Move whole leg front-up-back-down. Try to make two circles before lowering leg. After two circles, reverse direction, with left leg moving back-up-front-down. Begin with four circles in each direction and gradually work up to twelve. Reverse stem position and repeat movements with right leg.

MOVEMENT B:

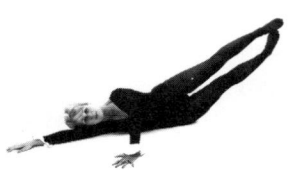

Lift left leg up and parallel to right leg. Hold position. Lift right leg up to meet left leg, until feet touch. Hold. Lower *only* right leg to floor. Continue to lift and lower right leg to left leg, which serves as the goal. For starters, lift the goal leg about two feet off the

The Hips 115

floor. As strength increases, lift goal leg higher. Reverse stem and repeat with right leg. Begin with four lifts to each side; increase gradually to twelve.

MOVEMENT C:

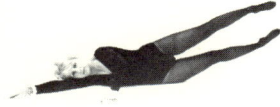

Lift left leg high off floor. Hold. Lift right leg up to meet left leg. Touch. Hold. Lower right leg to floor. Hold. Lower left leg to floor. The pattern is: Top leg up, bottom leg up. Bottom leg down, top leg down. Reverse stem and repeat with right leg. Begin with four; increase gradually to twelve.

MOVEMENT D:

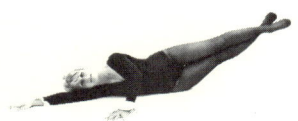

Let your left leg rest on right leg. Lift bottom leg off floor, carrying top leg as deadweight. Lift as high as you can. Hold. Return leg to floor. Repeat to other side. Begin with three lifts to each side; increase gradually to twelve.

STEM POSITION 2:

Kneel on hands and knees. Press insteps to floor. Head up.

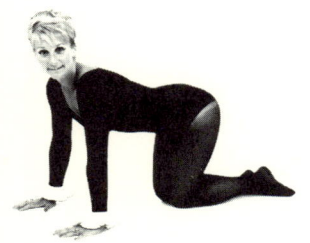

MOVEMENT A: 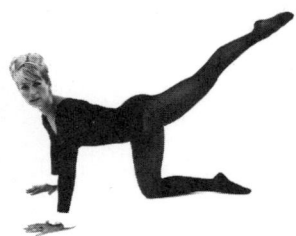 Straighten left leg back and lift it up as high as you can. Hold. Lower straight leg to floor until toes touch. Hold. Repeat high back lift five times on each leg; increase gradually to fifteen.

MOVEMENT B: 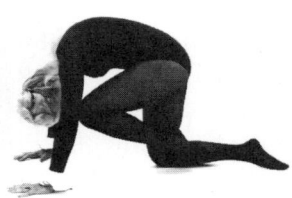 Bring left knee to nose as head lowers. Hold. Extend left leg back and up high, as head lifts. Hold. Repeat knee-to-nose and leg extension five times on each leg. Increase gradually to fifteen.

MOVEMENT C: 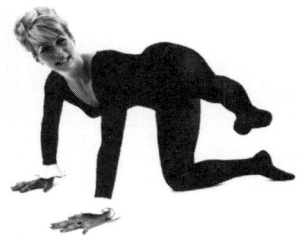 Extend left leg straight back, not higher than hips. Like a dog wagging a tail, swing left leg way around to left side, then back, and around to right side. It is a continuous movement. Keep leg off floor. Do not let it drag. Let your buttock and hip area wag right along. Begin with six on each leg; increase gradually to twelve.

The Hips 117

STEM POSITION 3: Lie on back. Knees bent to chest. Arms flat to floor, shoulder level. Palms down.

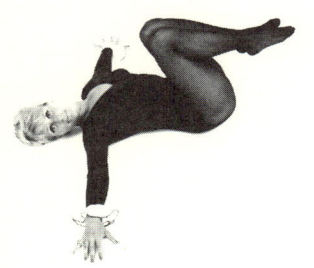

MOVEMENT A: Slowly roll both knees to right side. Hold. Return to stem. Roll knees to left side. Hold. Return to stem. Keep knees together. Try to slap thighs and knees to floor as you roll from side to side. Begin with eight; increase gradually to twenty.

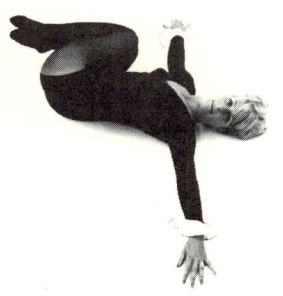

MOVEMENT B: Keep knees pressed together. Lower hip to right side, as in movement A. Hold. Slide knees up to touch right elbow. Hold. Release knees to stem. Lower hip to left side. Release to stem. Begin with eight; increase gradually to twenty on each side.

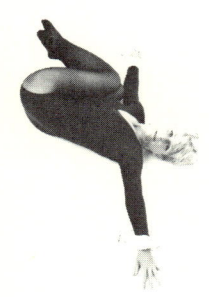

MOVEMENT C:

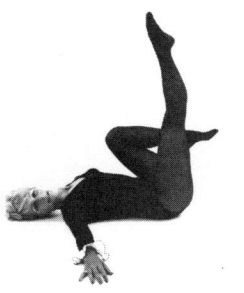

Extend right, then left, leg up toward ceiling. Start both legs moving in a vertical position, as if cycling. Let the motion carry into the hips. Begin with ten; increase gradually to thirty.

STEM POSITION 4:

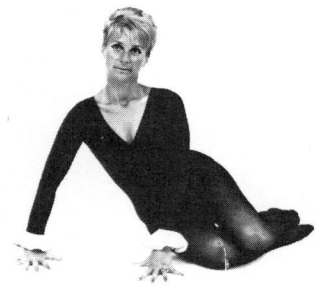

Sit erect on right hip. Legs bent together to right side. Hands resting on floor to right of knees.

MOVEMENT A:

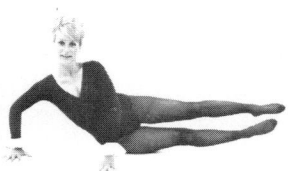

Quickly dart both legs straight out to left side. Complete a full stretch with both legs, left leg slightly parted and parallel to right leg. Hold. Bend both knees and snap them together to stem. Hold. Repeat six times to each side; increase gradually to twelve.

The Hips

MOVEMENT B:

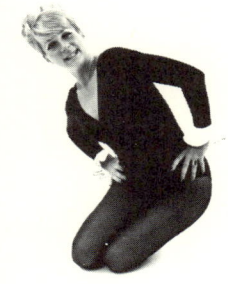

Place hands on hips. Roll buttocks up off floor and swing over to rest hips on left side. Hold. Swing buttocks to right side and sit on floor, resting on left hip. Hold. Continue to roll buttocks from side to side. Begin with four; work up gradually to twelve.

MOVEMENT C:

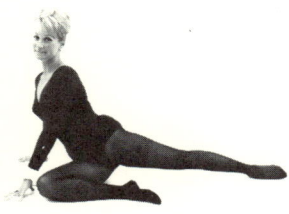

Extend left leg directly back until knee is straight. Toes pointed. Hold. Bend knee and slide leg back to stem. Hold. Begin with six while on right hip. Sit on left hip and repeat stretch with right leg. Increase gradually to twelve on each side.

STEM POSITION 5:

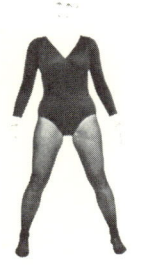

Stand erect. Feet apart hip width. Feet parallel. Arms relaxed at sides.

MOVEMENT A:

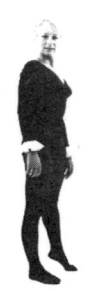

Keeping both legs straight, lift right heel high off floor. Hold. Lower heel to floor. Lift left heel off floor. Hold. Tense buttocks on each lift, release tension as hip lowers. Begin with six lifts on each side; increase gradually to twelve. For variety, lift and lower heel twice to each side, followed by four alternating single lifts.

MOVEMENT B:

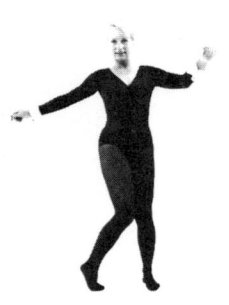

Place weight on left foot. Lift right heel off floor, keep right knee bent and turn right foot in, leading with the toes. Hip will lift up. Hold. Turn foot out, leading with toes. Heel is now turned in. Each time foot twists in and out, so does the hip. Try to twist as far as possible in both directions. Begin with ten to each side; increase gradually to twenty.

The Hips

MOVEMENT C: 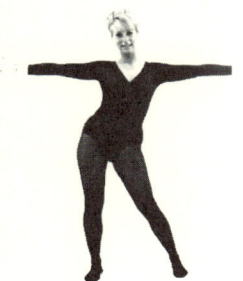 Extend arms to side, shoulder level. Without moving shoulders or chest, swing right hip way over to right side. Hold. Return hip to center. Hold. Swing left hip way over to left side. Hold. Return to center. Hold. Try to get hip to move freely in both directions. Do not bend knees. For variety, eliminate center hold; just swing hips from side to side. Begin with ten swings; increase gradually to thirty.

12 Area of Concentration: The Legs, Knees, and Thighs

The Problem. For every curve there is a muscle. And the curve is only as pretty as the muscle is firm and shapely. Thigh curves are four-dimensional because there are four regions to each thigh: front, back, inner, and outer. Your thigh problem may exist in one region, two regions, three regions, or all of them put together. This very much depends on your diet, work, and life-style. Unfortunately, I discovered in working with my patients that the exercises for inner thighs did not generally firm the outer thighs. It became necessary to develop specific exercises for all four thigh areas and to encourage my exercisers to use the proper ones for their individual problems. This is exactly what you will have to do.

If you're not sure where your thighs need attention, consult your mirror. Nude. Make a dispassionate appraisal of your thighs and use the appropriate exercises. You have nothing to lose but inches by trying them all.

The Program. The program is broken down to deal with all four trouble areas in the thighs. You will find exercises that will tighten the inside and outside of the thighs, slim your legs, reduce fatty knees, and generally restore a firm, attractive outline and strength to the entire area.

Technique Tips. The most important technique tip is the one that I have already mentioned. When you are lying on your back, always turn your head in the opposite direction from the working leg. This placement increases the stretch in your trunk and helps eliminate movements that might disturb your body placement.

Some of the exercises are labeled W. As in the arm exercises, this W means that they are designed to be done with weights if you wish to *increase* demands in order to hasten results. A one-pound weight on each ankle, or wearing skiing or hiking boots, will do the trick.

You will find when the stem position calls for a side floor position and your bottom leg is the anchor, bending the bottom leg slightly gives you more support and prevents rolling forward or backward during the movement.

EXERCISES FOR INNER AND OUTER THIGHS

STEM POSITION 1: Lie on right side. Head resting on shoulder and outstretched arm. Left hand flat on floor by chest for support. Legs straight.

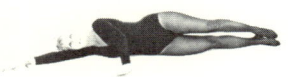

MOVEMENT A:
W

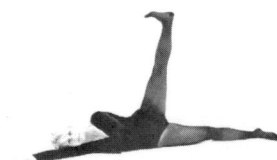

Slowly raise left leg high off floor, toes pointed. Hold. Flex and point foot four times in midair. Slowly lower leg to stem. Begin with six high lifts; increase gradually to twelve. Repeat on other side.

MOVEMENT B:
W

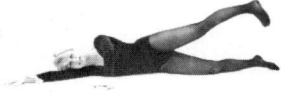

Turn left foot down with toes touching floor, heel turned up toward ceiling. Maintain this foot position. Lift and lower leg six times; gradually increase to twelve. Repeat on other side.

MOVEMENT C:
W

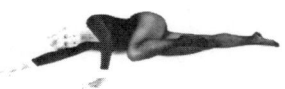

Bend left leg. Bring knee to left elbow. Hold. Extend leg straight out low, over right leg. Hold. Repeat. Continue bringing knee to elbow, then swiftly out straight. Begin with six; gradually increase to twenty. Repeat to other side. For increased action, pull knee under elbow, then straighten.

The Legs, Knees, and Thighs 125

STEM POSITION 2: Lie on back, legs extended toward ceiling. Knees straight. Arms flat to floor, shoulder level, palms down.

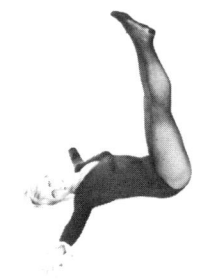

MOVEMENT A: Slowly separate legs as you turn toes toward each other. Imagine pulling a piece of taffy between your toes. Stretch legs apart as wide as possible, with toes turned toward each other. Hold widest position. Now, turn feet until toes point out to sides. Slowly bring legs together until heels touch. Repeat "taffy-pulling" stretch to widest position, then return legs to center until heels touch. Begin with four; increase gradually to twelve.

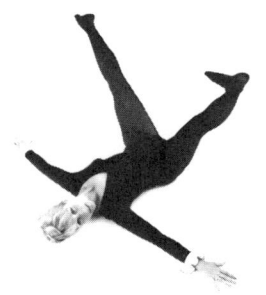

MOVEMENT B: Slowly lower left leg to left side until foot touches floor. Hold. Swing leg back to stem. Hold. Repeat with right leg. As leg lowers to either side, turn head in opposite direction. Keep leg straight and parallel to the arm. Begin with four; increase gradually to sixteen.

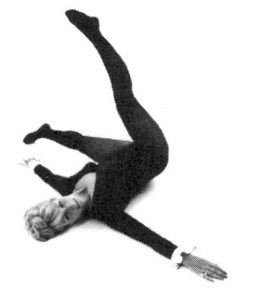

126   DOCTOR SOLOMON

MOVEMENT C:

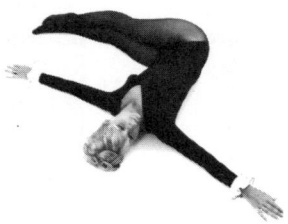

Slowly lower left leg to left side on floor. Hold. Lower right leg until resting on left leg. Hold. Release right leg to stem. Hold. Release left leg to stem. Hold. Repeat sequence to other side by lowering right leg to right side until foot touches floor. Alternate sides. Begin with four sets on each side; increase gradually to twelve.

EXERCISES FOR FRONT AND BACK OF THIGHS AND KNEES

STEM POSITION 3:

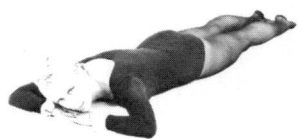

Lie on stomach, legs straight, insteps on floor, head down. Arms either under chin or extended front, palms on floor.

MOVEMENT A:

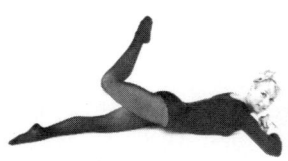

Lift right leg as high as you can. Hold. Bend knee, toes pointed toward your head. Hold. Straighten leg. Return to stem. Repeat with left leg. Begin with six; gradually increase to twenty.

The Legs, Knees, and Thighs

MOVEMENT B: Bend both knees on floor. Hold. With a moderate pace, and alternating, lift and lower each leg with bent knee. Lift as high as possible. Begin with ten; increase gradually to thirty.

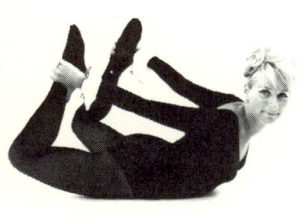

MOVEMENT C: Bend both knees. Reach back and grasp ankles firmly. Hold. Raise head, shoulders, chest, thighs off floor. Hold for two counts. Lower on two counts. When chin touches floor, repeat; do not release ankle grip until series is completed. Begin with three; increase gradually to twelve.

STEM POSITION 4: Stand erect. Legs wide apart, knees straight. Weight over center. Hands on hips. Or use one of the following aids: with both hands, hold back of chair or wall. Do not lean against aid.

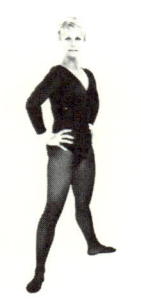

MOVEMENT A:

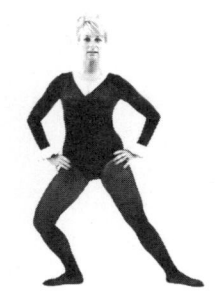

Bend right knee and lunge over right foot. Hold. Release to stem. Bend left knee, lunge over left foot. Hold. Release to stem. Anchor leg remains straight. Do not tilt trunk forward or backward. Begin with eight; increase gradually to twenty.

MOVEMENT B:

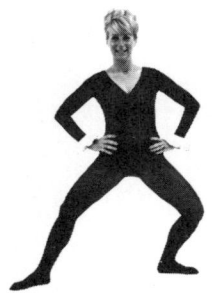

Bend right knee. Lunge over right foot. Hold. Bend left knee and shift weight over left foot. Hold. Stay in low lunge position and continue to shift weight from right to left leg. Begin with eight continuous lunges. Return to stem. Work up to sixteen.

MOVEMENT C:

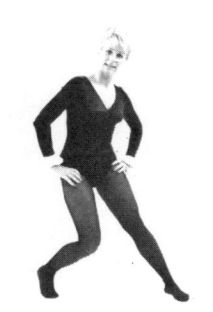

Turn right foot in toward center. Dip knee toward floor; as heel lifts up, keep left leg straight. Hold position. Return to stem. Repeat to left side, turning left foot in; knee dips almost to floor, heel lifts up. Hold. Release. Alternate sides. Begin with eight; increase to sixteen.

The Legs, Knees, and Thighs   129

STEM POSITION 5:   Stand erect. Feet together. Rest hands on back of chair. Keep arms straight.

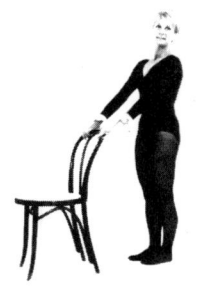

MOVEMENT A:
W

Lift right knee up to the outside of right arm at elbow level. Hold. Lower to stem. Alternate legs. Begin with ten; gradually increase to thirty.

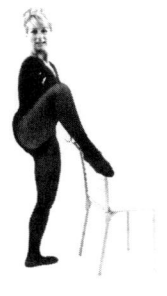

MOVEMENT B:
W

Bend right knee to chest. Point toes toward floor. Make circles with the lower leg, "can-can" style. Anchor leg remains straight. Begin with small circles, ending with big circles. Repeat with left leg. Begin with ten; increase gradually to thirty on each side.

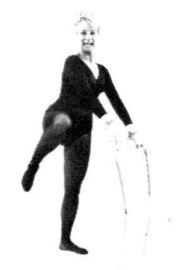

MOVEMENT C:
W

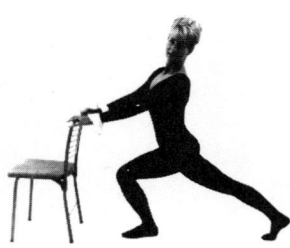

Lunge right leg directly back to full stretch, heel off floor, knee straight. Left knee bends. Try to press right heel to floor four times, keeping toes on floor. Return leg to stem. Repeat to other side. Alternate legs. Begin with four; gradually increase to twelve.

13 Area of Concentration: The Waistline and Midriff

The Problem. The reason I include the midriff together with the waistline is that the rib cage provides such a convenient hanger for fat. There it nestles, causing the midriff to expand and creep downward until there is a straight line from under the arms to the top of the hips. In fact, the problem is not one of the waistline, but one of no waistline at all. Scarlett O'Hara may have maintained a seventeen-inch waistline while eating like a field hand and doing nothing. But Scarlett had to be laced into a tight corset every morning, and I don't know a single one of my patients who would endure that for the sake of a waistline.

The Program. To replace a tight corset, I will show you how to awaken the muscles in the midriff-waistline area. As you increase the activity and stimulate the circulation, you'll notice that the inches go away without lacing. What's more, you'll have an advantage over Scarlett—your inches won't return every evening. This area responds beautifully to a program of bending, reaching, and twisting combined with proper diet.

Technique Tips. You will achieve a greater pull on your large areas during your stretches from either a floor or standing position by being careful of the way you hold your hands. Always have the raised hand palm upward. This produces a greater pull all the way down to your hips and buttocks.

When you are bending to the side or forward, don't use your arms or head for momentum. Instead, release your trunk upward by lifting first from the chest.

On side stretches, keep your movement localized by moving only the necessary muscles. Check your body position to be sure that you are not moving anything else.

Balance is essential in floor exercises, and you will find that the easiest way to maintain your balance is to be sure that your feet are properly aligned. If the stem says "Feet flat on the floor," press each toe on the floor. Flat means flat. This correct postural balance will give all parts of your body the opportunity to work together smoothly.

EXERCISES

STEM POSITION 1: Sit erect on floor. Legs wide apart and toes pointed.

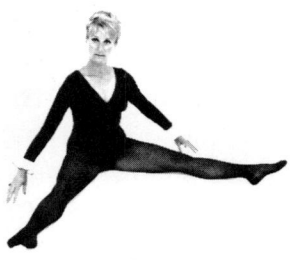

The Waistline and Midriff

MOVEMENT A:

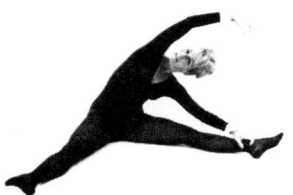

Grasp left ankle with left hand. Curve right arm over head, palm to the ceiling, and slowly bounce torso over left leg four times. Hold. Clasp hands over head and release trunk upright. Stretch up and pull waist off hips. Grasp right ankle with right hand; left arm curves over head, palm to ceiling. Slowly bounce torso over right leg four times. Hold. Clasp hands, release upright. Stretch and pull waist off hips. Chest faces front as you bounce over leg. Alternate sides. Begin with four and gradually increase to twelve.

MOVEMENT B:

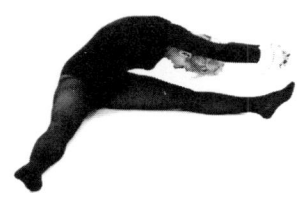

Clasp hands over head and turn upper trunk to left side. Slowly bounce over left leg four times. Try to touch hands to toes. Stop. Release to upright position. Turn trunk to right side and slowly bounce four times over right leg, trying to touch hands to toes. Release to upright position. Note that your chest is now facing your leg rather than open to the front. Alternate sides. Begin with four and gradually increase to twelve.

MOVEMENT C:

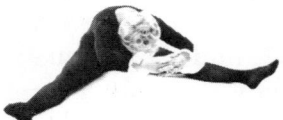

Clasp hands over head. Slowly bend deeply over left leg. Hold. Rotate trunk forward and over to right leg. Hold. Release trunk to upright position. Reverse direction and lower trunk deeply over right leg. Hold. Rotate trunk forward and over to left leg. Hold. Release trunk upward. Begin with four circles and gradually increase to ten.

STEM POSITION 2:

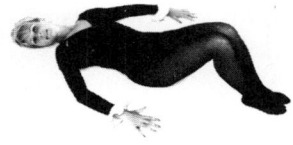

Lie on back. Knees bent and together. Feet flat on floor. Arms down at sides, palms down.

MOVEMENT A:

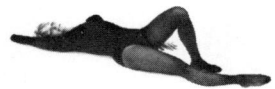

Simultaneously reach right arm back on floor as you stretch right leg forward, toes pointed. Stretch your leg and arm out as far as you can on the floor. Pull your waist off your hips as you stretch. Hold. Repeat long stretch to left side. Alternate sides. Begin with six and gradually work up to twenty.

The Waistline and Midriff 135

MOVEMENT B:

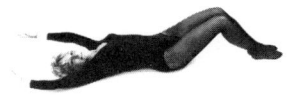

Lift both knees to chest. Hold. Keep knees bent and lower feet to floor, as arms stretch over head to floor. Hold. Lift both knees back to chest, as arms lower to floor. Hold. Repeat six times and gradually work up to twelve.

MOVEMENT C:

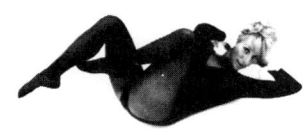

Lace fingers behind head at neck. Raise both knees off floor to chest as you lift head and shoulders up. Twist trunk and try to touch right elbow to left knee; then touch left elbow to right knee. Repeat four times. Slowly release feet and torso to stem. Begin with two sets of twisting and gradually increase to twelve.

STEM POSITION 3:

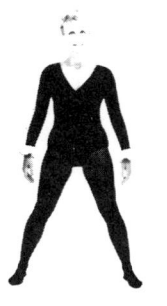

Stand erect. Legs wide apart. Knees over toes. Feet flat on floor. Arms down loosely at sides.

MOVEMENT A:

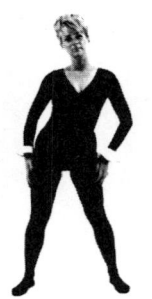

Without moving hips or bending knees, move rib cage (chest) as far to the right side as you can. Hold. Release to the center. Move rib cage over to the left side. Hold. Return to center. Move only your chest from side to side. If you have difficulty, practice in front of a mirror and place hands on hips to keep them immobile. Alternate sides. Begin with eight and gradually work up to sixteen.

MOVEMENT B:

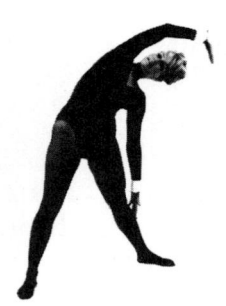

Curve right arm overhead, palm to ceiling. Bend deeply to the left side. Bounce over and try to slide left hand down leg toward ankle with each bounce. After four bounces, release slowly to stem. Repeat four deep bounces to right side. Be sure body bends directly to each side, neither front nor back. Begin with two sets of four bounces to each side and gradually increase to six sets.

The Waistline and Midriff

MOVEMENT C: Extend right arm out to side, shoulder level. Palm up. Keep arm shoulder level. Tilt head and stretch out to right side, bending at waist. Stretch four times over right arm. Release to stem. Repeat side stretch four times to left side. Begin with four sets and gradually increase to eight.

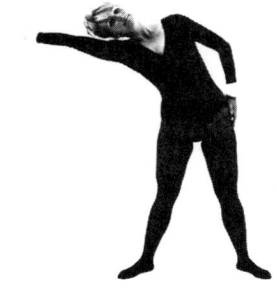

MOVEMENT D: Bend and try to touch right hand to the outside of your left heel. Hold. Release center. Repeat twist and try to touch left hand to outside of right heel. Begin with six and gradually increase to twelve.

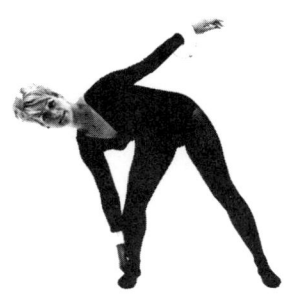

Part IV

14 Coping with Fatigue

How do you cope with fatigue? It's part of living, and it is also part of exercising. As I have discovered, it is certainly one of the excuses preferred by patients for *not* exercising. As I have also discovered, I can help my patients to cope with their fatigue in two ways: I can go to the root of the problem to discover if there is a medical reason for this overtired feeling (and in about 50 percent of the cases there is), or I can suggest some simple resting exercises to be integrated into the daily pattern that will alleviate much of the fatigue. In either case, whether the fatigue is physical or psychic, relief increases the ability to exercise.

It is important that you understand fatigue may be a warning of physical problems. Again, the best advice is to talk this over with your doctor to discover if this is the case. Whatever his decision, I am sure you will discover, as my own patients did, that using these resting exercises will help you cope with the fatigue.

The first two are positions for resting a painful back and are designed to reduce back strain. Just a few minutes in these positions can make a world of difference in your physical state and your mental outlook.

POSITION 1:   Lie on a bed that has a sturdy mattress. Turn on your side and pull knees up toward your chest.

POSITION 2:   Lie on your back in bed in a semireclining position. Prop up your knees with pillows until knees and hips are partially flexed.

Besides the above, there are three other resting positions designed to relieve back strain, neck stiffness, tension, leg ache, and general nervous tension. They may be done at home or at work.

HIP-FLEX REST   To relieve back strain and ache.

POSITION: Lie on back. Knees bent and together. Feet parted slightly, toes turned in toward each other. Arms resting relaxed at sides. Remain in position until you feel some relief.

SPINE RELAXATION: For when you feel tired all over.

POSITION: Put solid, straight-backed chair in a quiet place. Place mat or blanket on floor; have pillow nearby if needed to put under neck. Lie on mat with legs resting on chair seat so that knees are supported. The angle should be high enough for a mild upward hip-lift off floor. Relax arms at sides. Rest from five to fifteen minutes. Repeat daily as needed. If leg muscles are sore, place pillow on chair.

WORK BREAK: For relaxation and tension release.

STEM POSITION: Sit on a hard chair, feet flat on the floor. Feet apart, shoulder width. Arms down loosely between legs.

MOVEMENT A: Let your body drop until head is down between your knees. Your back should be rounded, arms and head dangling loosely. Slowly bounce toward floor (try to touch floor on third bounce), then uncoil slowly by pulling your body back up to the sitting position. Repeat exercise until you feel relief.

MOVEMENT B: When hands touch floor, hold position four seconds. Slowly uncurl spine until upright. Now stretch arms above head. Let your head drop back as you keep on stretching up and up and up until you yawn. Repeat forward drop and high stretch until you feel relief.

Enhance your resting times by following a few simple suggestions. These are most helpful if you feel the need of a breather between exercises, during any stressful times, or after sitting for long periods.

Allow yourself time to slow down. To induce a feeling of relaxation, try to make yourself yawn. Do not lie flat on your back unless you bend your knees in a hip-flex position; otherwise, you accentuate the curve or hollow in your back. Try to press the spine into the floor.

Curling and stretching movements are good for the spine as well as physically satisfying.

Relaxing on the floor with feet up on a chair or couch will help to renew your energy. It will allow the blood to flow more freely into your face, refreshing you in a short time.

15 Back Pain: Helpful Exercises

The Problem. Are you a candidate for backache? It seems to rank next after headache as a curse of civilization.

The back is a tension target, and pain there is a common complaint of both sexes of all ages. There are many causes for this, including the usual ones of overweight and lack of exercise. In addition to these, excessive strain on the spinal column, poor posture, and improper use of the back muscles when sitting, standing, walking, or bending will aggravate a swayback.

The Program: This chapter will teach you specific exercises to help you prevent back pain. You will learn explicit exercises to relieve the pain once it has started. Then you will finally find out how to care for your back every day to ensure its health and comfort—and your own.

Learning how to care for your back can minimize the frequency and intensity of any problems you may have had. Reducing the possibilities of backache is one of the most important and selfish reasons to exercise regularly.

Caution: If you are bothered with back problems right now, especially if you are in pain, consult your physician. Ask for his permission to do these exercises. *There are times when* no *exercise is best.*

When you have severe pain and muscle spasm in the back, it is most important that you remain in a comfortable, quiet position until the spasms cease. *If at any time during these exercises you feel an increase in pain, stop immediately.*

THERAPEUTIC EXERCISES

These four exercises begin with stretches, because stretching is effective in overcoming stiffness. These exercises also strengthen abdominal, back, and hip muscles. Start the exercises slowly and in the sequence indicated; this should allow the muscles to loosen up gradually.

The first three exercises start from the hip-flexed position on the floor or bed.

STEM POSITION 1: Lie on back, knees partially bent, feet together. Keep back flat against the mattress or floor.

MOVEMENT A: Lock hands together and cup over right knee. Pull knee slowly up against chest. Hold. Slowly return leg to original position. Repeat exercise with left leg. Begin with four knee presses on each leg; increase gradually to eight.

MOVEMENT B:	Lock hands together. Cup hands over both knees. Pull knees gently against chest. Slowly rock back and forth four times. This rocking creates a greater stretching effect on the tight muscles in the lower spine. Repeat this exercise four times and gradually increase to eight.
STEM POSITION 2:	Lie on side with both knees bent, head resting on pillow. Free arm rests loosely in front of chest.
MOVEMENT A:	Take a deep breath and relax. Slide upper knee toward chest as far as possible. Hold. Return to starting position. Hold. Begin with three knee-lifts to each side and increase gradually to eight.
MOVEMENT B:	Slide upper knee toward chest. Hold. Slowly lower leg until foot touches floor. Hold. Return leg to stem position. Begin with three full stretches to each side and gradually increase to eight.

When your back pain has completely subsided, you are ready to begin a series of exercises to help keep your back strong and healthy. However, for better back care, the preceding four exercises should be performed each time before the series of preventive exercises.

PREVENTIVE EXERCISES

This series of four exercises will teach you how to keep your back flexible and limber. It will also strengthen abdominal muscles while protecting the back.

Begin the exercises slowly and do them daily if possible. Use a rug or mat, and place a pillow under your neck if it feels better. Dress comfortably, removing shoes and socks or stockings.

STEM POSITION 1: Lie on back, knees bent, feet flat on floor, hands grip thighs. Keep stomach and buttock muscles tightened.

MOVEMENT A: *Note:* Keep chin tucked down on chest throughout entire exercise that follows as you come up (and down). Curl up as far as you comfortably can—to sitting position if possible. Hold. Slowly roll back to floor until shoulders touch. Repeat curl-up four times and gradually increase to eight.

MOVEMENT B: Repeat sit-ups, arms crossed against chest and hands gripping opposite elbows. Slowly curl up, then roll down. This variation increases the demands on the abdominal muscles. Begin with four and gradually increase to eight.

Back Pain: Helpful Exercises

MOVEMENT C: Repeat sit-ups with fingers laced behind neck. Slowly curl up, then roll down. This variation places even more demands on the abdominal muscles. Begin with four and gradually increase to eight.

STEM POSITION 2: Lie on back, right knee bent and foot flat on the floor, left leg extended on the floor. Arms rest at sides.

MOVEMENT A: Curl head, chest, and shoulders off the floor at the same time that you lift left leg off the floor. Bend leg toward chest. Grasp knee and try to press chin to knee. Hold. Slowly and simultaneously release leg and lower your upper torso to original postion. Repeat with other leg. Begin with four knee-chin curls to each side; increase gradually to eight. *Note:* Remember to keep the nonworking leg bent at the knee, foot flat on floor.

PROMOTING BETTER BACK HABITS

How many times a day do you unknowingly contribute to a backache? Doing your everyday tasks properly should help avoid the type of stress that causes back pain.

Do you always carry packages, books, groceries, or a briefcase in the same hand? It is better to shift loads from time to time from one hand to the other.

When you drop something, do you bend over to pick it up without bending your knees? If you keep your knees straight, you strain your lower back. Lift properly: bend both knees before you stoop, thereby involving your thigh muscles, not those in your back. Never lift anything above your chest, if possible, and always keep the load close to your body. Pushing an object higher than the shoulders forces an arching of the back, which causes strain.

Do not stand in one position for long periods of time with both knees straight. When you do, your hips sag forward and the back arches. Avoid this when you can. Bend one knee by placing the foot on a stool or box. This position tends to flatten the back and reduces the chances of back fatigue. If it isn't possible to elevate your foot, shift your weight from one foot to the other periodically.

Many of us sit still for long periods of time at a desk, piano, or sewing machine. We tend to hook one foot under our body, or slump to one side. Think about your sitting posture at work. A chair too high for your legs will increase back sway, because the knees are then lower than the hips. Try to keep knees higher than hips by placing feet on a stool or sturdy box. You should also support your elbows on the arms of your chair. Check your office chair. Replace it, if you can, when it is too high for you, or if it has no arms.

Add up the number of hours you spend in a car. Give some thought to your posture there, too. Do not sit far away from the pedals. The flexing of the knees is important here. Move the seat comfortably closer so that legs are not fully extended.

Poor sleeping posture often leads to restless nights. It is best not to sleep on your stomach. This causes the trunk to sag into the mattress with the back arching. Lying flat on the back increases a tendency to swayback. If you must sleep in this position, bend your legs and stack pillows under the knees. Optimum position for your back is to lie on one side with hips and knees bent, curled up into a ball. I strongly recommend a firm mattress, no matter what your position.

Weight control has a direct relationship to back fatigue. The smaller the waistline, the fewer pounds your body carries around, and the better the chances for alleviating back strain.

Think before you move. Utilize daily the tips suggested above. They may help to relieve your backaches. Remember that incorrect sleeping and sitting habits, as well as inactivity in everyday life, may contribute to back-muscle fatigue. Ask yourself: Will this position give me a pain in the back?

16 On the Road

Keep on moving. Like dieting, exercise expertise must be *maintained.* In a society of people who restlessly surge from one spot to another for business or pleasure, I have discovered that there are days containing too little time or space for the Master Plan.

At first I inclined toward sympathy. Since I must travel myself, I realize the restrictions travel places on people. However, human beings share certain traits, and I came to realize that permission not to exercise while traveling soon extended to the days before travel and the days after travel—and there I would be with a patient who had ceased to exercise.

The solution was obvious, a *mini* Master Plan of five *maintenance exercises* that could be performed in the limited time and space of the traveler. They are also great for days when the world at home closes in on you, because wherever you are, these exercises are designed to overcome stiffness and loss of muscle tone. Their most important function, however, is to keep you in touch with your exercise commitment until you can resume full-time activity.

My patients have come to call these their "everywhere" exercises. I was surprised to learn that many of them practice these in addition to, rather than as a substitute for, the Master Plan. One of my patients reports that this is an ideal break in her housework, and one of my dieting secretaries has substituted an exercise break for her ten-minute office coffee break.

Wherever you are, if you have a belt, a towel, three feet of cord, a rolling pin, or a stick, you will find these good aids during these exercises. My sister, Evalee, reminds me that whenever she travels she takes along a jump rope; between trips it is conveniently left in her suitcase.

The Problem. The problem, in addition to keeping muscles flexible when there is no time for the Master Plan, is to help relieve some of the tensions of travel.

The Program. The program is one of bending, stretching, and rotating the body. It is designed to keep you limber, not to replace your regular exercise program. This is a reliable *substitution* to fall back upon on the rare occasions when you are limited to a lesser activity.

If you have back problems, check with your doctor before using these exercises.

POSITION:	Stand erect, with legs wide apart, knees relaxed, and feet front. Place exercise aid across your shoulders and hold firmly.
MOVEMENT:	Slowly bend forward from the hips, keeping your head up. Bounce low toward the floor four times. Slowly release to an upright

position. Repeat the low bounce. Return to an upright position. Begin with five and gradually increase to twelve daily. *Note:* If your body is stiff, bend your knees slightly as you bounce.

BENEFIT: For flexibility, as a stretch and general conditioner.

POSITION: Stand with legs apart, knees relaxed, and feet front. Hold exercise aid firmly behind body, arms straight.

MOVEMENT: Bend forward from the hips until chest is parallel to floor. Keep your head up. Slowly lift exercise aid up and away from your body. Keep lifting. Hold. Lower exercise aid to body and straighten up. Repeat high lift, then begin again. Begin with six and increase to twelve.

BENEFIT: Firms upper arms, shoulders, bustline, and chest.

POSITION: Stand tall, with legs wide apart, knees straight, and feet firmly on the floor. Place exercise aid behind neckline and hold firmly.

MOVEMENT: Slowly twist upper torso to the right until looking directly behind you. Hold. Return to center. Repeat full twist to the left side and hold. Return to center. Twist only at the waist. Keep back straight. Do not tip forward or back. The more you twist, the easier it becomes. Begin with six and increase to twelve.

MODIFICATION: If troubled with a weak or bad back, pivot on sole of left foot by lifting your heel off the floor as you twist to the right. Repeat modification, with your right foot pivoting as you twist left.

BENEFIT: Slims waistline and develops freer body movement.

POSITION: Stand erect, with legs wide apart, knees relaxed.

MOVEMENT: Pull abdominal muscles in tightly. Bend forward from your hips with your head up. Take four swim strokes forward with your arms, keeping abdominal muscles held tightly. Stop. Stand erect and release abdominal muscles. Repeat exercise four times. *Note:* Do not hold breath while holding abdominal muscles in.

BENEFIT: Strengthens and firms abdominal area.

POSITION: Stand erect, with legs apart and feet turned out. Hold exercise aid overhead, arms straight.

MOVEMENT: Slowly stretch upper torso to the right side as you bend your left knee, and lunge over your left foot. Hold this "opposition stretch" for two counts. Release and straighten to center. Repeat opposition stretch to the left side, bending upper torso to the left side as you bend your right knee and lunge over your right foot. Hold and then release to center. Begin with six and increase to twelve daily.

BENEFIT: Improves body tone and flexibility. Firms hips and thighs.

17 Family Fitness

Why pay the fees for your family to trek to a gym or spa for a physical-fitness program? Your home is perfectly adequate as a physical-fitness center. You have the devices you need right at hand for exercise aids. Of course, right now they are masquerading as household implements; but with a little imagination, I know that you can discover their true purpose.

For example, weights. If you want to exercise with weights, as I suggested previously, there are many one-pound weights right on your pantry shelves. Check out those cans you have stacked there. Most of the vegetables are sixteen-ounce cans, and that's a pound weight.

Just because you are dieting, don't throw out your rolling pin. Convert it to more healthful purposes by using it to help you in your waistline-stretching exercises. Once you've swept your floor, turn your broom into an exercise wand as you bend and twist to trim your midriff.

A strong motivation for joining a gym or spa is the social one. I realize that many people do find it easier to exercise when they have company. So why not involve the company whose health is most important to you? Gather your family together for a family-fitness program. In days when the sociologists are decrying the fact that families fragment their activities, you can outwit the doomsayers and outwit the health statistics by involving everyone from the toddler to grandma and grandpa in an activity program.

Here's how to do it. Have equipment available at all times of the day. As I said, use your imagination when it comes to equipment. When your family has become more engrossed in the program, it may be worthwhile to invest in aids that keep their interest alive. At the outset, however, they will be intrigued at the thought of using a can of beets in one hand and a can of pineapple in the other as weights.

Set aside an exercise corner. It can be in the den or recreation room if your house is large enough; otherwise, a corner of a bedroom or bath is perfectly adequate. Be realistic, and you will find that there is very little expense involved. All that is really necessary is a slant board (which can be your ironing board), a jump rope, broom handles for each family member (why not spray-paint each a different color?), two full sixteen-ounce cans, and a six- to eight-inch rubber ball. This minimum amount of equipment takes up very little space in any closet; in fact, there is a compact unit designed to go on the back of a closet door for the purpose of holding ironing equipment that will keep this exercise equipment very neatly.

Set your record player or tape system up so that it is readily available to your exercisers. You may not be into rock, but if rock is what will keep your children working out with you, my advice is to learn to love it. It's a great beat for exercising.

If I came along and promised you that I could help your children to do better in school and at their extracur-

Family Fitness   159

ricular activities, that I could assist you in making housework easier, that I could show your husband how to unwind at home and at work, and that I could top this off by improving family communications, you would probably be very skeptical. Yet this is exactly what I can do for your family, if you will follow through on my suggestion that you exercise together as a family group. I firmly believe that one of the most important benefits of this program is the family interaction, because it promotes family mental health.

So for physical *and* mental health, let's begin with some group exercises.

GROUP EXERCISES

Here are some fun exercises for the entire family. Pick a leader who will give instructions and count out loud for the group. The number of repetitions can be determined by the energy and fitness level of those participating.

STEM POSITION 1:   Lie on back on floor in "chain" formation. Arms out straight at shoulder level. Each person holds the wrist of the person beside him, keeping arms taut.

MOVEMENT A: Lift right leg up high. Hold. Lower leg to right side, foot touching floor. Hold. Swing leg across body to left side until foot touches floor. Return leg to center, then lower to floor. Repeat leg swings with left foot. *Note:* Everyone should try to keep arms and shoulders firmly on floor and must move in unison.

MOVEMENT B: Slowly lift both legs high off floor. Hold. Keeping legs together, lower legs to right side until bottom foot touches floor. Hold. Return legs to center. Hold. Lower both legs to left side. Hold. Return to center. Lower legs front to floor. *Note:* Keep shoulders pressed firmly to floor. Work in unison.

STEM POSITION 2: Everyone sits in a circle, legs crossed at ankles. Place hands on shoulders, elbows front. Pick a leader.

MOVEMENT A: Slowly, as a group, drop heads to chests. Lower until elbows touch floor. Hold. Leader decides how many counts group stays in low curl position. Upon signal, slowly uncurl to original position.

STEM POSITION 3: Stand and make a circle. Hold hands. Legs together.

MOVEMENT A: Simultaneously step forward, lunging on the right leg, knee bent. Hold. Left foot remains in place. Return to stem position. Lunge forward on left leg. Hold. Return. Arms swing forward with each lunge, then lower on return. *Note:* Hold hands throughout exercise.

This next group of exercises is especially beneficial for the younger members of your family. Children love rhythmical, challenging activity, and you can be the one who introduces your children to this delight. Before your children are exposed to school gym classes, you have the opportunity of developing their flexibility, motor skills, and confidence within the family unit. I can imagine no greater joy for a child than this introduction to exercise, having fun with the family and receiving praise and encouragement for achieving along with the adults. It should promote a feeling of closeness and enjoyment for all.

BALL STRETCHES

STEM POSITION 1: Sit on floor, legs together. Place ball on floor by right hip. (Use any rubber ball six to eight inches in diameter.)

MOVEMENT: With right hand, roll ball forward and around feet over to left side, then behind body. Change hands and continue making a circle with the ball by rolling it first with the right hand and then with the left (in the opposite direction). Try to keep knees straight. Variation: Separate legs on floor, head front, and try to roll ball all around body. Try to keep knees straight!

STEM POSITION 2: Sit on floor, legs straight and parted slightly. Place ball between legs at ankles.

MOVEMENT: Lift both legs off the floor, tossing ball free as legs separate. Catch ball before it bounces to floor. Replace ball between straight legs, at ankles. Repeat lift-toss.

STEM POSITION 3: Stand with legs wide apart, bending forward from hips. Ball is centered between legs, on the floor.

MOVEMENT: Take ball in right hand as right knee bends in a lunge. Pass ball behind right knee to front, as left hand receives ball. Lunge to left side, pass ball with left hand behind knee around to the front. Continue to lunge and pass ball behind each leg several times. *Note:* When one leg is bent, the other is straight.

STEM POSITION 4: Stand with legs together. Hold ball in either or both hands.

MOVEMENT:	Bounce the ball and turn yourself completely around before catching it and before it bounces a second time.

Do not be surprised if your children are more agile at some of these exercises than older members of the family.

PARTNER EXERCISES

Working together with another member of your family in partner exercises is also a good exercise in learning how to adjust to another's personal skills and limitations. It provides another area in which those emotionally close to one another can learn more about each other's personalities. Even in the happiest families, I feel that this simple aid in getting to know one another better can produce new and better relationships.

When you establish a set time for being together and exercising together, rain or shine, you are saying that what you are doing as a family to keep everyone happy takes precedence over the outside world. You are providing this for your children and for your other family members because of everyone's deep concern for the others' health and well-being. So pair off and begin these:

STEM POSITION 1:	One person sits on floor, legs wide apart, knees straight, toes pointed. Hands resting on floor, palms up.
MOVEMENT:	Stand behind partner. Place your hands firmly on sitting partner's shoulders and gently press shoul-

ders forward toward floor. Floor partner aids in bounce by moving from hips, and rounding back. When floor partner feels limber, change positions.

STEM POSITION 2: Both partners sit on floor facing each other tailor fashion, legs crossed at ankles. Arms extended to sides at shoulder level, palms forward. Distance between partners may have to be adjusted once exercise is begun.

MOVEMENT: Each partner twists to his left until right hands touch. It is important to keep the back and both arms straight throughout twist. Sit far enough apart to make each twist a stretching challenge.

18 Sexual Fitness for Men and Women

When it comes to exercise that is fun, the all-time favorite is undoubtedly sex. It burns a fair number of calories, 200 per couple per incident. Naturally, if you want to increase your calorie burning, you must increase your sexual activity. Sex is a mystic mingling of the spiritual and the physical. One of the most pleasant is to liberate yourself by liberating your mind. Learn how to turn yourself and your partner on to sensuality. Evalee's movement therapy classes have given her clients a heightened sexual awareness through the following exercises.

CREATE SOME SENSUOUS PLEASURES:

. . . Invest in some silky sheets and always store them with scented sachet. As you turn and move, the currents of air will waft sweet scents about you.

. . . Have a pair of his and hers caftans for you and your partner to wear. Let the softness of the material caress your bodies as prelude to your lovemaking.

. . . Think about the evening when you dress for the day. Wear minimal underwear—if any. As a surprise for your mate, when you strip away your daytime clothes, wear a sheer bikini and seethrough bra, or, for men, colorful French-cut briefs.

. . . Create a mood by drinking from long-stemmed wine goblets before an open fire with some incense or a scented candle burning.

. . . Bathe together by candlelight in a luxuriously scented tubful of warm water. Or shower together, but at a languorous pace, soaping and rinsing each other gently and lovingly.

. . . For the ultimate in all-around sensation, make love on a furry rug with comfortable squashy decorative pillows around to use as sexual props.

. . . Take an air bath nude before an open window with the breeze titillating your skin. (Just be certain that your open window opens where there are no prying eyes.)

. . . Keep a large, movable mirror in your bedroom.

. . . Learn the art of massage so that you can relax each other into sexual desire through tender, loving care.

. . . Play background music of your choice so that even your ears participate in your sex.

Now, having learned to create the mood for sexual activity, you can also create a body that is physically able to enjoy sex totally. I have some very simple exercises that will liberate your body, just as mood-setting liberates your mind. Think about the words "awareness," "ability," "agility" in terms of your sex life. Are you inadequate in any of these vital areas? Specific exercises will help you stimulate a variety of movements and rhythms to enhance your sexual pleasure.

As you acquire the ability to shift the various parts of

your body, your confidence and ease will increase. You will want to use this new liberation to experiment and enjoy new sensuality and self-expression.

The first five exercises are presented from a strictly sexually functional point of view. The last one is a favorite of everyone who tries it because it is a sensuality warm-up for men and women. This may be the most important chapter of the book for your overall lifetime enjoyment. No more bedroom blues after you have learned and practiced these exercises. You may want to practice to background music that suggests the sensual beat of the tropics—bongo or conga drums, or the slow, undulating *taxim* in belly-dancing music.

The Problem. During a discussion of exercise, Ms. K. said that her husband complained of her lack of agility whenever they made love. "Every time I try to be agile," she said, "I end up with leg and foot cramps, really severe charley horses. It's very hard to be sexy when you can't move your legs."

The Program. The way to eliminate the charley horse is to become limber enough to be naturally agile. You can increase your flexibility in bed, as Ms. K. did, with the following exercise. Practice it today, and then try it again tonight!

STEM POSITION 1: Lie on your back. Legs together, straight and extended toward the ceiling, toes pointed. Arms extended to sides, shoulder level.

MOVEMENT A: Place hands inside thighs by knees. Slowly and gently press legs apart. Keep knees straight. When widest position is reached, continue to gently press legs apart. Hold for eight counts. Slowly draw legs together to stem position. Repeat several times daily. Begin with a series of three; increase gradually to eight.

MOVEMENT B: Without help from hands, repeat wide leg stretch. In widest position, begin to flex feet. Flex heels on "one," point toes on "two." Continue to flex, point both feet while stretching legs farther apart. Begin with six flex stretches; increase gradually to twelve.

MOVEMENT C: Without hands, repeat wide leg stretch, toes pointed. Find widest comfortable position. Hold two counts. Turn knees out. Slowly draw legs together until soles and heels firmly touch. Keep knees wide apart. Hold two counts. Straighten legs and release to wide-open position. Repeat four times; gradually increase to twelve. Slowly release to stem position. *Note:* To rest between variations, slowly bend knees to chest.

Results. "Well, let me tell you, this exercise was quite a turn-on, not just for me, but for my husband too. I never knew such sensations existed, and I've been married fifteen years. I can get my legs up and into many different positions that I never dreamed of, because they are stronger. I can hold the positions, too, with no cramping of my style!" That's a direct quote from Ms. K.

The Problem. "My problem is my hips," was Ms. B.'s complaint. "I seem to be so constricted in this area that I know it has to affect my sexual activity. Can you help me?"

The Program. What I suggested to Ms. B. is an exercise that is made to order for this problem. It is a pelvic lift combined with rhythmic hip-tilting. By doing this exercise, you learn how to control your body through isolating the hip and pelvic area. The best way to do this is in tempo with your earthiest record; and if you don't have one, buy one so that you learn to move to it.

STEM POSITION 2: Lie on back. Legs wide apart. Knees bent feet flat on the floor. Arms extended out to sides, shoulder level. Palms down.

MOVEMENT A: Slowly, to the count of four, lift hips off the floor. Hold. Try to lift pelvis higher on four more counts. Hold. Slowly lower hips to stem position on four counts. Rest. Begin with four lifts and increase gradually to eight.

MOVEMENT B: Slowly, on four counts, lift hips high off the floor. Hold. Lift only *right* hip up and down from this position, four times. Your left hip will lower slightly during the action. Then lift only the *left* hip up and down four times. Each time you lift your hip up, let it drop naturally to your uplifted position. Lift hip up on "one," drop on "two," up on "three," drop on "four." The hip movement should be slow, deliberate, and powerful. Slowly lower to the floor and rest. Begin with four and increase gradually to ten.

MOVEMENT C: Slowly, on four counts, lift hips high off the floor. Hold. In this uplifted position, make a complete circle with your hips. After three circles to the right, lower hips to the floor and rest. Repeat three circles to the left. Keep stomach flat during circles. Begin with one set of hip circles and increase gradually to three sets.

Results. When I spoke to Ms. B. later that month, she told me that she was like a different woman in the bedroom. "I didn't recognize *me* in bed . . . and he didn't either! I'm moving my body around differently because I feel much more confident and my rhythm has improved."

The Problem. Mr. M. came to me with this request: "Do you have a suggestion for me for an exercise? I'm athletic and in good shape until it comes to sex. Sometimes before sexual activity my whole body goes limp and kind of relaxed; and even though I am inwardly excited, this feeling overwhelms me."

Sexual Fitness for Men and Women

The Program. My suggestion for Mr. M. was that he prepare his body for this intense activity just as he would for any of his other athletic events, by warming up the muscles he was going to use. The program consists of contracting and then releasing the buttock muscles. This slow, rhythmic tightening and releasing of musculature as a prelude to and during intercourse is a great help. It increases stimulation and excitation for many men, and it eliminates the body limpness that bothered Mr. M.

STEM POSITION 3: Lie on stomach. Chin resting on hands. Insteps flat to the floor.

MOVEMENT A: Slowly, on four counts, squeeze your buttocks together by tightening and tensing those muscles. Hold them together for four slow counts. Slowly release on four counts. Do not hold your breath. Repeat entire sequence four times and increase gradually to eight times.

MOVEMENT B: Quickly, on one count, draw buttock muscles together tightly. Hold them taut for two counts. Quickly release on one count. Continue this quick contraction and release five times and increase gradually to ten. Then *slowly* draw buttocks tight. *slowly* release.

Results. Mr. M. summed up the results in one word, "Terrific!" Then he went on to say, "Just practicing this muscle contracting made my initial thrust so much more intense that it increased pleasure for both of us. Now I even have more control of my body during intercourse. By the way, my wife uses these exercises also and it has increased her muscle agility too. We love the extra pleasure it affords both of us!"

The Problem. "My problem is certainly not desire," admitted Ms. C. "That I have, but I am very short on ability. There's no problem when it comes to the basic position, but I'd love to vary this with a 'side-to-side' or something more exotic. When I try, I find that I am very uncomfortable. Quite frankly, I'd like a little of the spice of life that variety brings. Can you help?"

The Program. I had an exercise for Ms. C. that is called the hydrant. It is guaranteed to teach you how to move and adjust your body in unfamiliar ways. With practice, you will find that the exercise has prepared you for the variety—and the spice—that Ms. C. so ardently desired.

STEM POSITION 4:	Kneel on hands and knees. Insteps flat on the floor. Head up.
MOVEMENT:	Keep right knee at same kneeling angle and lift leg up high to the right side, level with shoulder. Hold high elevation two counts. Return leg to bent-knee floor position. Begin with five lifts on right side, then five on left side. Gradually increase to twelve lifts on each side.

Results: Ms. C. could not wait to call me with the

news. "This was the funniest exercise I have ever tried. I exercised my face muscles from the first lift of my leg, I was laughing so hard. It's just what I wanted; I've added so much stretch and strength to my legs that I can do almost anything in bed!"

The Problem. I suppose every man alive has heard and told some variety of the wife's headache joke. Well, as a male I must confess I hesitate to divulge the next complaint from a man for fear that it will let loose among the women a new family of jokes dealing with their husbands' backaches.

While I was discussing exercise as part of his weight-reduction problem, Mr. R. took advantage of the conversation to say: "Every time I have sex, I pay for it with low-back pain a few hours later. My weakest lovemaking muscles are obviously in my back; and while they don't bother me during the act itself, it sure as hell is inhibiting to know that in two hours' time I'm going to hurt. And I wouldn't mind one bit if any exercise you gave me increased the amount of time I could spend making love. I mean, if you've got a good thing going, why not keep it going?"

The Program. My advice to Mr. R. was to strengthen his back and leg muscles in order to increase his sexual fitness.

STEM POSITION 5: Sit on the floor with hands on the floor behind buttocks. Stretch legs wide apart.

MOVEMENT A: Slowly raise buttocks off the floor. The hands and heels will support body during the lift off the floor.

Hold uplift for two counts. Slowly lower buttocks to floor. Begin with five lifts and gradually increase to ten.

MOVEMENT B: Repeat the body lift. While in midair, thrust pelvis back and forth rhythmically several times. Slowly lower to floor. Repeat five times and gradually increase to ten.

Results. Mr. R. reported back in the following month with the happy news that back pain and inhibitions were things of the past. Not only that, he said he found that the position and movement fulfilled his other request as well. Mr. R. is one man who found everything he needed to know about sex along the way to losing weight and toning up. He now enthusiastically recommends diet and exercise to all of his friends—and so does his wife.

Finally, here is the sensuality warm-up I promised you.

SPECIAL SENSUALITY WARM-UP

STEM POSITION 6: Lie nude on your back on the floor. Legs wide apart. Arms stretched beyond head on floor, and relaxed, palms up. Drape a silky transparent scarf across your body.

MOVEMENT A: Slowly raise pelvis and rest of body off floor. Press heels to the floor for support. Hold for two counts. Slowly return to the floor. Repeat body uplift and rhythmically perform a shimmy motion from left to right with your hips until scarf falls off. From time to time, vary the tempo and hold a position momentarily for dramatic effect. Repeat movement until you feel pleasantly breathless.

MOVEMENT B: Repeat body lift with one leg crossed over the other at the ankle. Try to keep legs and thighs tightly *squeezed* together, and repeat pelvic shimmy from left to right until scarf shifts on your body, revealing more of you. Repeat as often as you desire.

19 Exercising Eating Awareness

There is a natural progression in going from the subject of sex to the subject of eating. Eating can be a voluptuous experience. For many, it is superior to sex, and that is truly a problem. However, if my patients learn to exercise eating awareness during the period when they are reducing and exercising, I find that the problem of maintenance very nearly solves itself.

Just what is eating awareness? Eating awareness is being conscious of each mouthful of food taken in, from the moment it leaves the plate until after it has been swallowed.

Medical and psychological studies have shown that overweight people eat more quickly than the nonobese. Thin people seem to have developed techniques to control the speed at which they eat. They have either an inborn or an acquired sense of pace.

This is most important, because medical data have shown that it takes approximately twenty minutes after eating for the brain to receive a message from the stomach of being filled—that feeling of satiety. That is why mealtime should be leisurely. The slower your process of eating, the less you will eat. When travelers return from Europe with tales of meals that last two to three hours and families that eat this way daily without being obese, that is the explanation.

You can learn to slow down your eating behavior by learning to inhibit a quick response to food. You can learn not to gobble and gulp. I shall suggest some specific exercises in eating awareness that you can experiment with. Select the ones that work for you or develop your own variations. Your own individual preference and life-style will determine how you should exercise to obtain eating awareness.

I. EXERCISING CONTROL

1. To counter tension before you eat (because many dieters *do* feel apprehensive as mealtime approaches), try some self-relaxation techniques. Breathe deeply and fully. Relax all of your major muscles, starting at your head and working down through your toes. Stretch your body fully and slowly.
2. Once you are seated at the table, make a ritual of unfolding your napkin and having a sip of water, stalling the actual first eating movement for at least one full minute.
3. After the first bite of food is in your mouth, concentrate on chewing slowly and deliberately. Chew thoroughly before swallowing.
4. Before you take a second mouthful of food, be sure that you have swallowed the first.
5. Place a mirror on the table so that you can watch your eating movements. You may be thoroughly surprised to see yourself in action. This single exercise has alerted many of my patients to what they were doing and effectively motivated them to change their eating habits.
6. Build delays into your meals by: pausing between bites,

spending longer between courses, and placing your utensils on your plate after each mouthful until it has been chewed and swallowed.
7. Talk a lot about pleasant things, but only with an empty mouth.

The next section contains eating exercises that we have taught successfully in obesity workshops. These break down the eating process into its components. As you become aware of each one, you will slow down your eating, find the process more pleasurable, and eat in moderation.

Practice the following exercises whether you are eating alone, with your family, or with someone special.

II. EXERCISING EATING AWARENESS

1. Concentrate on your breathing, not on the food.
2. Close your eyes and slowly inhale the scent of the food.
3. Take time with chewing. Chew the first bite thoroughly on the left side of your mouth, then swallow. Chew the second bite thoroughly on the right side, then swallow. The third bite, chew your food on one side, pass it to the other side, and chew it there before finally swallowing. Repeat this process with each three bites of food.
4. Roll food around in your mouth. Run your tongue over it. Press it up into the roof of your mouth. Coat your mouth with the food.
5. Hold the food in your mouth for several seconds.
6. Experiment with different-sized bites of food.
7. Practice a conscious awareness of every bite that you eat. This will keep you constantly aware that you must eat slowly.

Does all of this work? I can say with certainty that it does. Not only do my patients and Evalee's clients become aware of the way they are eating and what they are eating, they make other discoveries as well.

Some of the discoveries are very simple. I had one patient who found out that for years she had chewed only on the right side of her mouth. Why, she had no idea, but learning to chew on both sides bestowed new sensations of flavor and satisfaction on the simple act of eating her food. She enjoyed eating so much more that she automatically slowed down—the very purpose of the exercise.

For another of my patients, Ms. D., French bread had been an enormous part of her overweight. She gobbled it by the loaf. Then I insisted that she slow down, roll the bread around in her mouth, and really investigate it for taste and texture with her tongue. She was surprised to realize that the reason she had always gobbled French bread so quickly was not that she liked it, but that she *didn't* like it at all. For years she had been eating it as fast as possible to get it out of her mouth. The discovery liberated her from thousands of extra calories.

Another patient, this one a man, slowed his eating down and found that he could not eat slowly. He needed dental work, and eating quickly had masked the effect of hot and cold foods on his sensitive teeth. Awareness of eating forced him to the dentist's office to obtain the physical relief that he needed. Then he could, and did, eat slowly.

You see, what you learn from this exercise may be useful in more ways than one. It is tremendously important for you to explore your real relationship to the food that you eat. By slowing down the pace of your eating with this combination of control technique and mastery of eating exercises, you can not only increase your enjoyment of food by savoring each mouthful, but can also learn to eat less because you are conscious of what you are eating.

Eating behavior is an important part of any weight reduction program, and learning to modify poor eating behavior is on an equal footing with learning about good diet. As assistant professor of psychiatry and behavioral science at Johns Hopkins School of Medicine, I have been aware of the link between both aspects of weight loss for a long time.

Last year the Diet Workshop introduced behavior-modification techniques into its group weight-control program. What the organization discovered in the first year of working on eating behavior has borne me out. As I write this, other group weight-control organizations are about to add exercises in changing eating behavior to their programs. Now *you* have the basic techniques in the forms of specific exercises.

Once you begin practicing these exercises, I am sure that you will uncover much about your eating habits that you had buried away.

The final one is the old but true one: when you have finished eating what is before you, the best exercise of all is to place both hands firmly on the edge of the table and push yourself away before you take any more.

20 Movement Therapy

Perhaps a more accurate title for this chapter would be "Movement *as* Therapy." Movement can be therapy for unused body parts. Almost everyone settles into a groove, either because of work or because of general life-style. Once the groove is established, physical activities become programmed, the range of body movement is restricted, and the muscles respond by wasting away. It sounds very dull and self-defeating, and it is.

The awareness quiz that you took back in Chapter 3 was to make you cognizant of your particular groove—of where your movements are restricted. That's a most important exercise in itself: Simply becoming aware of what parts of your body are frozen, and why. Climbing out of grooves takes effort. It takes *movement.*

The purpose of this chapter is to prescribe movements as a therapy for the dullness and self-defeat of your grooved day-to-day activities. We want to evoke within each of you a response to your bodies and an awareness of them. We want you all to experience the creative sense that planned movement bestows so that you begin to use your body as an expressive tool. Rather than repeat the same restricted motions, you will do the same tasks with a difference. More muscles will take part. Your walk, your posture, your involvement, and your appearance will change. You will find that days seem different because you no longer permit them to be monotonous. Living is more fun when you move actively through life.

You can be as creative as you want. There is no right or wrong way to move. You are the one who determines what is right or wrong for you. By indulging in these movement activities, you will feel different about yourself. You will want to change some of your activities because you have learned that your body responds happily to new demands on it. The more of your body you move, the more your body will appreciate it.

MOVEMENT-THERAPY ACTIVITIES

PROBLEM AREA: Frozen shoulders.

SOLUTION: A movement activity to discover a new or different way of moving your shoulders.

POSITION: Lie on back, knees bent, feet flat on floor and together, arms out to sides with palms to floor.

MOVEMENT: While keeping hands and elbows pressed to the floor, try to lift both shoulders up off the floor. Hold two counts. Release shoulders to floor. Repeat movement several times, until you begin to feel a freedom in your shoulder movements. Then repeat shoulder lift by alternating each shoulder.

PROBLEM AREA: Frozen rib cage and chest.

SOLUTION: A movement activity to free your rib cage and chest area.

POSITION: Lie on the floor on your back. Find a comfortable position. Imagine that your chest is a large paintbrush.

MOVEMENT: Moving only your chest, begin to paint the ceiling. Let your movement grow larger and try to paint as much of the ceiling as possible. Explore different strokes with your chest brush. Try dabbing and flicking movements; long, short, and circle strokes. Continue to body-paint until you feel satisfied that you are beginning to unfreeze your chest area.

PROBLEM AREA: Frozen neck.

SOLUTION: A movement activity to extend your range of neck movements.

POSITION:	Sit on the floor, legs crossed at the ankles and eyes closed.
MOVEMENT:	Turn head slowly until chin is over left shoulder. Slowly, with the tip of the nose, write your full name from left to right. Use as much space as possible. Stop. Using your chin and moving from right to left, erase your name, using as much space and head movement as possible. Repeat several times until you feel your neck loosen and the movement feels comfortable.
PROBLEM AREA:	Frozen hips and pelvis.
SOLUTION:	A movement activity to involve the pelvic region.
POSITION:	Kneel on the floor on your hands and knees, with your knees shoulder-width apart. Lace fingers tightly, with palms pressed to the floor. *Do not remove hands from the floor or even shift their position.*
MOVEMENT:	Leading with your hips and pelvic area, try to move your body in as many different ways as you can; try swaying, twisting, bumping,

etc. Experiment with different levels. In time, you can invent different ways to move by working around this imitation. The more you work with your pelvic and hip area, the freer it will become.

When Evalee first introduced these movement exercises, some of her clients were slightly hesitant to try them. Even though they practiced them in private, she could sense a certain reserve and self-consciousness about the procedure, because at first they did not understand the reason behind the exercises.

However, as the weeks passed, there was a change in attitude along with a change in the range of the individuals' movements.

You may have many of the same reservations. Well, lots of things we do in life appear silly if we view them dispassionately. So are a lot of the postures we assume in ordinary actions. Why should movement therapy be any different?

Try these exercises seriously and systematically. It is a *liberation program* for your muscles, your body, and you. Call it a muscle revolution, if you will, but throw yourself into it, for the results are long-term and beneficial.

Once the thaw sets in, your frozen body parts will move you through any room with more style and grace.

21 How to Relax

As we move through life we also move through periods of stress and tension. I can imagine nothing more boring than a life that involved no tension or stress. I think most of you would agree. Still, we all require some assistance in dealing with periods when stress and tension seem to be largest part of the day. The best assistance I can offer you are some self-relaxation techniques to counteract the harmful effects which hectic periods of your life may bring about.

Does this have anything to do with exercising and weight loss? Of course it does. Obese people counteract their tensions by overeating. It's the way they have learned to cope. Then overeating adds to the stress just as soon as they realize what they have done, because it causes guilt feelings. And so they react to the new stress as they did to the original one—by overeating. Stress and tension are also concerned with exercise. The body reacts to emotional tension with physical tension. Exercise brings muscles into play that dissipate the physical tension; and sometimes this acts to relieve the emotional tension as well. At the very least, exercise will make you aware of your body and its muscles so that you may participate more freely in the act of auto-relaxation.

For those who know that tense situations will bring about compulsive behavior such as overeating or excessive smoking, I suggest self-relaxation as a deterrent to other acts like opening a box of chocolates or filling an ashtray with cigarette stubs. Substitute a constructive act for a destructive one.

Relaxation is a deliberate action, one that you learn through a set of patterns. Once you have learned these exercise patterns, you have them for life.

Self-relaxation is based on three elements: *deep and slow breathing, concentration,* and *imagery.* I have four patterns for you to learn. You may use them separately or in sequence. I find these patterns work if people practice them twice a day until the response becomes automatic. Just repeat each pattern until you feel relaxed.

At first, while you are learning, you must have *a calm environment, a comfortable position,* and *a passive attitude.* That's a tall order for someone who has a life-style of stress. I guarantee it's worth the effort to find the triple combination—either at home, or at work, or while traveling.

Find a comfortable chair that supports your arms and your head. If it is more comfortable for you, lie on the bed or floor. Remove your shoes and loosen any tight clothing.

Remember, you are *learning.* Don't worry about achieving a deep level of relaxation. Just concentrate on one of the patterns from the four suggested. Rid yourself of any unpleasant thoughts or concerns by imagining a big jar, sweeping the unpleasantries into it and, in your mind, capping it. You can deal with those matters another time.

PATTERN 1: Find a comfortable position in a quiet environment. Close your eyes slowly. Listen to the rhythm of your breathing. Inhale through the nose in one long breath. Exhale through the mouth. Take twice as long to exhale.. Each time you exhale, try to prolong your exhalation. Keep lips slightly parted and your jaw relaxed as you exhale.

PATTERN 2: Find a comfortable position in a quiet environment. Close your eyes and listen to the rhythm of your breathing. Place a hand on your body where you feel your breath coming from. If the hand is higher than your navel, your breathing is shallow. Replace your hand slightly below your navel. By placing your hand below your navel, your breath will respond to touch and you should be able to breathe more deeply.

PATTERN 3: Find a comfortable position in a quiet environment. Close your eyes and listen to the rhythm of your breathing. Inhale through your nose, and imagine your breath starting from your toes and flowing up the entire front of your body to your head. Exhale. Imagine your breath flowing down the back of your body to your toes. Continue to imagine that your breath circulates up the front and down the back of your body.

PATTERN 4: Find a comfortable position in a quiet environment. Close your eyes and listen to the rhythm of your breathing. Imagine three uninflated balloons connected to each other in your body, one below the navel, one in your chest, one in your head. Slowly inhale through your nose and fill up each balloon with your breath. Imagine your breath flowing first into the navel balloon, then into the chest balloon and finally into the head balloon. Exhale, and deflate each balloon one by one from the top down.

Afterword

The best prescription I know of for my body is *movement*. When I am feeling good and move, I feel better and more alive. When I am feeling low and overburdened, movement lifts me out of myself to a new level of energy and hope.

For me, the *now* of movement is the best tonic that I can recommend, and I hope it can be for you, too.

Glossary

A list of terms frequently used to explain various exercise movements and positions demonstrated in this book.

ANCHOR: Nonmoving part, referring to a leg or hip.
BOBBING: To bounce or move up and down.
BOUNCE: To bob or move up and down.
CONTRACT: Muscle tensing, to draw muscles together.
CURL: A slow lifting or lowering of the trunk. (a) Curl up: in order of head, shoulders, chest, spine lifting up. (b) Curl down: reverse this order.
DIAMOND PATTERN: Soles and heels pressed together, knees out to the sides.
EXTEND: To lengthen, to lift, to straighten.
FLAT TO FRONT: *See* Square.
FLEX: To bend, to press at right angles, *i.e.*, hand to arm, foot to leg.
GRIP: To clench; as in clench toes—to curl toes under.
HIP-FLEXED POSITION: Knees together and bent, feet flat on floor.

HOOK: Floor position. Sit on right hip. Right leg bent, knee pointing front and on floor. Left leg bent, with left knee pointing out to left side on floor. Left foot on floor behind body. Reverse for other side.

HORIZONTAL MOVEMENT: Denotes a level or direction of movement. Parallel to the floor or body.

INSTEP: The arched middle portion of the foot.

LACE: To interlock—usually refers to the fingers.

LATERAL: Side; side sections.

LOCK: To tighten; to render immovable, to keep in place; such as to tighten knee by straightening leg.

LUNGE: To step far out on one foot, knee bent and supporting most of your weight.

PARALLEL: Side-by-side position or movement.

PRONE: Face-down position.

RELEASE: To relax, to let go, to return.

SQUARE: To keep the chest directed front. Right shoulder to right wall, left shoulder to left wall.

STEM: Original position or movement.

SUPINE: Lying on the back.

SWEEP: To make a continuous and extending (curving) movement; to cover the entire area.

TAILOR FASHION: Sitting position on the floor, to cross legs at ankles with feet under knees.

TORSO: The trunk of the human body.

TUCK: To pull in or together; to squeeze; to tighten; to pinch in.